The **Can Do** Multiple Sclerosis
Guide To Lifestyle Empowerment

Patricia Kennedy, RN, CNP, MSCN, has been working in the field of MS since 1987. As a nurse practitioner at a comprehensive MS center in Denver, Colorado, her role has been providing neurologic care for hundreds of people living with MS. She has been part of the professional staff of Can Do MS for 24 years and more recently joined the office staff as well. In addition to working with people individually, she spends much of her time speaking to professionals involved with the treatment of MS as well as people with MS and their partners throughout the United States and Canada. She is active in the International Organization of MS Nurses and has helped mentor many of the MS nurses in practice today. She serves on committees of the National MS Society and is active in The Consortium of MS Centers. Her passion for MS comes from working with people who are able to see beyond the limitations and uncertainty that the disease brings and move on in their lives in a direction that enhances a better quality of living. She has recently relocated to Virginia to be closer to her children, grandchildren, and the beach.

THE **CAN DO** MULTIPLE SCLEROSIS
GUIDE TO LIFESTYLE EMPOWERMENT

EDITOR
Patricia Kennedy, RN, CNP, MSCN

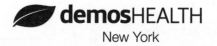

New York

Visit our website at www.demoshealth.com

ISBN: 978-1-9363-0318-2
e-book ISBN: 978-1-6170-5081-7

Acquisitions Editor: Noreen Henson
Compositor: diacriTech

Medical information provided by Demos Health, in the absence of a visit with a health care professional, must be considered as an educational service only. This book is not designed to replace a physician's independent judgment about the appropriateness or risks of a procedure or therapy for a given patient. Our purpose is to provide you with information that will help you make your own health care decisions.

The information and opinions provided here are believed to be accurate and sound, based on the best judgment available to the authors, editors, and publisher, but readers who fail to consult appropriate health authorities assume the risk of injuries. The publisher is not responsible for errors or omissions. The editors and publisher welcome any reader to report to the publisher any discrepancies or inaccuracies noticed.

Library of Congress Cataloging-in-Publication Data

The can do multiple sclerosis guide to lifestyle empowerment / editor Patricia Kennedy.
    p. cm.
    Includes index.
    ISBN 978-1-936303-18-2
    1. Multiple sclerosis—Popular works. 2. Self-care, Health—Popular works. I. Kennedy, Patricia, 1942–
    RC377.C32 2012
    616.8′34—dc23

2012013706

Printed in the United States of America by Hamilton Printing
12 13 14 15 / 5 4 3 2 1

Dedicated to Jimmie Heuga:
our inspiration

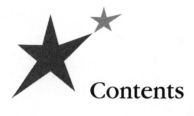

Contents

Contents

Contributors

Peggy Crawford, PhD, is a Clinical Psychologist at UC Physicians, Department of Neurology, University of Cincinnati, Cincinnati, Ohio. Dr. Crawford's training and clinical experience as a health psychologist over the past 20 years have afforded her the unique opportunity to work with and learn from individuals and families living with MS. She has had the privilege to share in the life stories that define the journey over the course of MS and has reflected these stories in presentations, research projects, and publications. As a member of the Can Do MS professional staff for 8 years, she has formed meaningful collaborations and connections with other professionals as well as individuals with MS and their families. These relationships have nourished her passion for working in the field of chronic illness just as time in Maine has nourished her soul.

David Engstrom, PhD, ABPP, is a Clinical Health Psychologist, on the medical staff of Scottsdale Healthcare, Private Practice, Scottsdale, Arizona. With over 25 years of experience working with people with MS, Dr. Engstrom has served as a psychologist at Can Do MS programs for many of those years. After receiving his PhD from The University of Southern California, he was on the faculty at the University of California, Irvine Medical School. He has now relocated from California to Scottsdale, Arizona. Dr. Engstrom has authored many publications in health psychology and has an active schedule of public speaking. In addition to his passion for helping people with chronic illness and weight management, his other primary interests are motivational coaching, stress management, and sleep disorders. In his spare time, he enjoys spending time with family, hiking, running, fly fishing, African hand drumming, and Tai-Chi.

Barbara S. Giesser, MD, is a Clinical Professor of Neurology, David Geffen UCLA School of Medicine, Los Angeles, California. As a neurologist, Dr. Giesser has specialized in the care of persons with MS for 30 years. She is a New Yorker by birth, a Texan by training, and currently a Californian by geography. She received specialty training in MS under the direction of Dr. Labe Scheinberg at the Albert Einstein College of Medicine. She has authored books on the subject of MS and lectures to professionals and people living with MS and their partners. She has had the privilege of working with Can Do MS for almost twenty years. In addition to her academic credentials and accomplishments, she is very proud to have briefly been a technical advisor on *The West Wing*.

Rosalind Kalb, PhD, is a Clinical Psychologist at the National Multiple Sclerosis Society and a proud member of the Can Do program staff since 2004. As a clinical psychologist, Dr. Kalb has specialized in MS throughout her 30-year career. After 20 years as a staff psychologist at an MS comprehensive care center, she joined the National MS Society in New York. Roz is the senior author of *Multiple Sclerosis for Dummies, 2nd ed.* (Wiley Publishing), co-author with Nicholas LaRocca, PhD, of *Multiple Sclerosis: Understanding the Cognitive Challenges* (Demos Health), and the editor of *Multiple Sclerosis: The Questions You Have—The Answers You Need*, now in its 5th edition, also from Demos Health. When she's not pursuing her interest in MS, Roz is busy enjoying the beauties of Maine with her husband, the very same Nick LaRocca.

Patricia Kennedy, RN, CNP, MSCN, is a Nurse Educator at Can Do Multiple Sclerosis, Edwards, Colorado. Pat has been working in the field of MS since 1987. As a nurse practitioner at a comprehensive MS center in Denver, Colorado, her role has been providing neurologic care for hundreds of people living with MS. She has been part of the professional staff of Can Do MS for 24 years and more recently joined the office staff as well. In addition to working with people individually, she spends much time speaking to professionals involved with the treatment of MS as well as people with MS and their partners throughout the United States and Canada.

Sue Kushner, MS, PT, is Director of Clinical Education at Slippery Rock University, Slippery Rock, Pennsylvania. Sue Kushner has been a practicing physical therapist for 25 years, working in academics and the clinical setting. She combines her knowledge of exercise physiology and her passion for exercise and yoga when working with patients or teaching. Sue has done volunteer work for the National MS Society locally and nationally for 23 years and has been on the Can Do MS staff for 22 years. She resides north of Pittsburgh with her two teenage children.

Ann Mullinix, OTR/L, is currently working as an Occupational Therapist at Methodist Hospital/Park Nicollet, St. Louis Park, Minnesota, where she works with an adult population in an outpatient setting. Ann has worked as an occupational therapist in a hospital clinical setting in Minneapolis for 23 years and for 19 of those years has also been as a professional staff member of Can Do Multiple Sclerosis. Ann began working with Can Do MS while she was working with Randy Schapiro, MD, and his MS team in Minneapolis. Ann's specialty areas include neurological rehabilitation and development of visual perceptual/cognitive treatment. Ann devotes her personal time to her family— husband Scott and three teenaged children—mentoring single mothers, and implementing preventive injury training programs for young athletes.

Baldwin Sanders, MS, RD, LDN, is an Assistant Professor in the Department of Health Sciences, Western Carolina University, Cullowhee, North Carolina. where she teaches nutrition and health courses. She earned a Masters in Public Health Nutrition from Columbia University, and has previously taught at Louisiana State University and the University of California at Berkeley. She has worked as a nutrition consultant with Can Do MS for the past 17 years. She enjoys lecturing on nutrition and MS, individual counseling to improve health and well-being, and the complementary alternative medicine aspect of nutrient supplementation with MS. She lives with 3 goats, a pig, numerous chickens, roosters, a turkey, 3 rabbits, 3 dogs, and a cat.

Randall T Schapiro, MD, FAAN, is President of The Schapiro Multiple Sclerosis Advisory Group in Eagle, Colorado, and Clinical Professor of Neurology, Retired, at the University of Minnesota in Minneapolis. Dr. Schapiro has been involved in the team approach to multiple sclerosis for over forty years, and founded one of the first comprehensive MS Centers in a private practice setting in 1977. While that center remains active in Minneapolis, he has retired from practice but continues to teach nationally and internationally about MS to those with the disease as well as those involved in care of MS. He was a founding member of the Consortium of MS Centers and has received the Can Do award from Can Do MS. As a person interested in athletics, he has been a "runner" for over 35 years, served many years as the neurological consultant for *Runner's World* magazine, the Minnesota Twins, and the Minnesota Vikings. He coached his kids through their youth baseball and basketball careers.

Andrea White, PhD, is an Exercise Physiologist and Research Associate Professor at the University of Utah, Salt Lake City. Dr. White has been involved in MS research for over 15 years, examining exercise effects and factors influencing fatigue. Her ski racing background provided a special connection to the community of Can Do MS, and she participated in and organized Snow Express for MS fundraising events for over a decade, as well as serving as a Staff member for the Can Do MS program. She recently was awarded the Jay Gurmankin Volunteer of the Year Award from the Utah-Southern Idaho Chapter of the National Multiple Sclerosis Society for her service as Research Advocate and Clinical Advisory Committee member. A believer in an active lifestyle, she is an avid cyclist and continues to ride for MS every year.

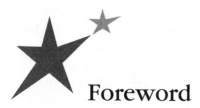

Foreword

Living with a chronic disease is not easy. It must be especially difficult after making extraordinary physical achievements by the age of nineteen. I can't imagine the daily challenges faced by those diagnosed with multiple sclerosis (MS). But I can tell you that choosing to live life fully, regardless of the hand you are dealt, is what my father, Jimmie Heuga, did the best.

Some of the most vivid memories I have of my father are of his striking smile and long, strong hands. These are what I still see when I reminisce and have wistful father-daughter chats these days.

These are the same hands that tightly gripped me as we rode T-bars up the ski slopes in the late 1960's, and that consoled and guided me through so many of the important decisions in my life. As a child I worshipped my dad. He took me everywhere, like a leash-less puppy, as I stumbled all over myself trying to please him. If he had to leave me for a couple of hours to teach skiing, he'd pin a note on me that said, "If lost, please return to Jimmie Heuga at the ski-school hut." We seemed to always be laughing, playing, or testing each others' similar stubborn streaks.

Dad was raised with strong core values and a diligent work ethic that supported his belief that attainable goals are always within reach. His "Can Do" perspective guided him early on through Olympic skiing success and continued through the unknown waters of a lifetime of living with MS. Despite the unpredictable changes in his health over the years, Dad met those challenges with a positive attitude, and as a family we adjusted along with him. We followed his lead by matching his enthusiasm with our own. When he had to start using a walker for mobility, we decorated it with ski stickers. When he moved to a wheel-chair, we put snow tires on it. Dad walked his talk by believing passionately that everyone with MS can live a full and satisfying life.

Each chapter in this book is thoughtfully written by members of the Can Do MS staff. These individuals are experts in the field of MS care management and are dedicated to the life philosophy my Dad pioneered. The information provides a foundation to help create a personal lifestyle strategy to meet the unique challenges of living with a chronic disease. This book provides tools you can use to take control of your life, especially when facing an uncertain future.

So read on. I know that regardless of how your life is touched by MS, you will find help, support, and empowerment in the pages that follow.

Kelly Heuga Hamill
Board Member
The Jimmie Heuga Center Endowment

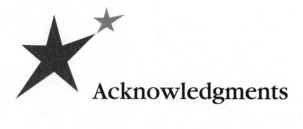 Acknowledgments

We wish to acknowledge the entire program staff of Can Do Multiple Sclerosis. Without this team, our message of empowering people living with MS and their support partners to be more than their MS would go unheard.

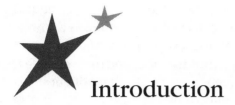

Introduction

WHAT IS CAN DO MULTIPLE SCLEROSIS?

In 1964, as Jimmie Heuga won the Olympic Bronze medal for downhill skiing, he did not know what his future held. He was absorbed in the moment of winning an Olympic medal and sharing his tremendous accomplishment with family and friends. It wasn't until he was diagnosed with multiple sclerosis (MS) six years later that his future became uncertain.

Jimmie often told the story of sitting in his apartment after being diagnosed with MS, and looking at all of the people who were exercising and participating in recreational activities. He had been advised to avoid such activities, which was standard medical advice at that time. However, as he looked down at the active people he began to feel a sense of loss. After a brief period of self pity, he made a decision about his future: he was going to resume an active lifestyle. As an athlete, an active lifestyle was a very large part of who he was and how he was raised. If it was, in fact, harmful, as suggested by the medical community, he would at least enjoy the time and stop feeling sorry for himself. At that point, he asked his landlord if he could borrow a bike. After borrowing the bike, he hopped on it, rode a little, lost his balance, and fell. He got back on, rode a little more, lost his balance again, and fell. This repeated itself many times until Jimmie found himself miles away from his apartment. What he realized at that moment was that he had ridden the bike and forgotten about the diagnosis of MS. His concentration was on staying upright and not falling. Now that he was miles from home, he was more concerned with how to get back than the fact that he had MS. Most importantly, he felt a sense of normalcy and stopped his negative feelings. He went on to resume his exercise program with a sense of purpose and realized this was having a positive effect on the way he felt, both physically and mentally. For Jimmie, this created a lot of questions about the advice he had received concerning exercise and MS. It also created a lot of questions for his loved ones who were seeking answers. Could he be the only one who would experience these benefits from exercise? Could exercise actually be good for people with MS?

Jimmie did not have all the answers about exercise or living with a chronic disease like MS, but with the hope of maximizing his quality of life, he felt the best thing for him was to resume what he knew best. He began to question local medical professionals about his experiences with physical activity, and he surrounded himself with like-minded people in the medical profession and other experts in MS management. That led him to better define his future by founding an organization to further explore his personal experiences through interactive programs and research. In 1984, The Jimmie Heuga Center was founded, and it continues today as Can Do Multiple Sclerosis (Can Do MS).

The fundamental principles of Can Do MS remain the same as when it was founded in 1984. As Jimmie discovered, he was able to draw a distinction between the value of attending to his overall health as opposed to totally focusing on living with a chronic disease like MS. Today, Can Do MS continues to work with people and families living with MS to draw that same distinction. As in 1984, there is no cure for MS. However, unlike 1984, there are multiple treatments available to manage the disease and symptoms, allowing people with MS to remain active. As medical advances found more options to treat the disease of MS, ongoing treatment shifted from one of managing relapses and symptoms to managing the disease. This was a very exciting advance for people living with MS. However, there was still a need to educate people about strategies to manage their health along with their disease. What started as a program solely focused on exercise for people with MS quickly grew to programs that provided a wide range of strategies to help people identify their "anchor," much as Jimmie identified his anchor as his exercise program. Jimmie's exercise program became his "personal GPS," guiding him through his uncertain journey with MS.

Over the years, lessons have been learned from the thousands of people with MS and their families who have participated in Can Do MS programs. Health care professionals who have shared their expertise during those programs have learned as well. In 1984, Jimmie's ideas were seen as revolutionary, but they have stood the test of time. Can Do MS programs and services continue to be unique in how they are delivered, with an emphasis on a family-centered approach and proactive management of health and disease.

A fundamental premise of Can Do MS is that individuals need to contribute to their health and quality of life through identification, achievement, and communication of goals to their health care team. Likewise, health care providers need to listen to their patients with MS and openly communicate with them. It is this bi-directional communication that helps maximize treatment and quality of life when living with a chronic condition such as MS. You will hear throughout this book the importance of establishing a health care team. MS can affect everyone differently, and therefore, utilization of different members of a health care team may be required at different times. Knowing how and where to access these professionals is essential. Each member of the team has a unique point of view. Contribution to overall care and the ability of those health care professionals to communicate and coordinate treatment is extremely advantageous. In many cases, the person living with MS will need to play a major role in that communication and coordination process.

Another important lesson learned over the years, and often emphasized by Jimmie, is that there will be ups and downs and successes and failures as a person moves through their MS journey. Jimmie often said that he "never set a goal that didn't knock him on his butt." He used those experiences to evaluate, re-set his goals, and start again. This is an important principle to keep in mind while reading this book and starting to identify goals.

This book aims to provide a foundation for helping the person with MS to be in charge of their health care. The book can act as a "personal GPS" by helping you choose a plan. There are usually many different ways to set a course, and sometimes there are detours on one course requiring a switch to another path or direction. This book can serve as a guide that you can revisit in order to program or re-program that GPS. Everyone is different and each approach is unique. Therefore, the suggestions provided will be different based on the information needed for the journey. Throughout the book highlighted questions will ask: *What Can I Do?* which will help and encourage taking control of the different aspects of health and health care. Just as Jimmie did not know his future when facing the diagnosis of MS, everyone can have uncertainty that can be worsened by the diagnosis of MS. We hope this book can provide a foundation to help lessen some of that uncertainty and promote better health.

LIFESTYLE EMPOWERMENT

Everything we do at Can Do Multiple Sclerosis is driven by one simple belief: You are more than your MS. With a vision, a mission, and core values rooted in the legacy and belief of our founder, Jimmie Heuga, that everyone living with MS has the power to live full lives, Can Do MS is the start of a whole new way of thinking about and living with MS.

Lifestyle empowerment is about learning the individualized skills and mindset to take charge of your health and your life with MS. Lifestyle empowerment is about helping you regain a sense of control, dignity, and freedom by teaching you and your support partner how to overcome your unique challenges and create a personalized lifestyle.

Can Do MS's whole person, whole health, and whole community approach to MS provides people with MS and their support partners with a deeper and broader understanding of their unique condition. It explores the physical, interpersonal, emotional, intellectual, and spiritual aspects of living with MS. By gaining more in-depth understanding of their unique condition, their body, and themselves, and blending that knowledge with realistic and personalized goal setting, individuals learn what is possible with MS, and how to live fuller, richer lives within the constraints of MS.

SETTING GOALS

Each of the chapters in this book deals with a different aspect of the whole person, whole health, and whole community approach to living with MS. Start off by reading the Motivating and Goal Setting chapter. This chapter will teach you how to plan for your goals. Then read each subsequent chapter with these goal-setting concepts in mind. When you find an area in which you need or want to set a goal, refer back to the Motivating and Goal Setting chapter. For example, when you read Eating Well, Eating Easy, you might discover that you would like to set goals around healthier eating. Refer back to Motivating and Goal Setting to assist you in creating your plan to eat healthier.

HIGHLIGHT AND UNDERLINE STRATEGIES

This book is chock full of useful strategies and ideas. To keep these strategies fresh in your mind, you might find it useful to mark up this book. Feel free to highlight or underline strategies that you would like to refer back to at a later date. You can do this with a print version or most e-readers. Another suggestion is to get a sticky notepad and mark specific pages you would like to refer back to.

WHAT CAN I DO?

This book provides a foundation for helping you be in charge of your health care and helping you discover that you are more than your MS. Throughout the book, highlighted questions will ask: *What Can I Do?* Asking and answering these questions will help and encourage you to take control of the different aspects of your health and health care.

We hope this book can provide a foundation to help determine what you *can do* to maximize your health and quality of life, and discover the power to be more than your MS!

The **Can Do** Multiple Sclerosis
Guide To Lifestyle Empowerment

1 Motivating and Goal Setting

David Engstrom

How can you change your habits and health behavior in lasting ways? Both goal setting and proper planning are excellent methods to keep motivation alive. In reality, all people set goals for themselves, many times, only to see them unfulfilled. Why does the very admirable act of setting a goal often have a disappointing outcome? How do we get off track? The material and exercises in this chapter will help you to learn and practice some simple and efficient methods for establishing goals and plans that will be more likely to keep you on track.

USE THIS CHAPTER AS AN ANCHOR

Read this chapter first and get a grasp of how to plan for your goals. Then read each subsequent chapter with these goal-setting concepts in mind.

TRY EXPERIENTIAL LEARNING

"It's all in the doing." In order to get motivation and set goals, the first move is always to *do something different*! Behavior change, no matter how small, is what causes motivation, not the other way around. You can't get motivation just sitting on the couch! Whenever we change our behavior, our attitudes toward that change become more positive. In other words, every time you read about a useful strategy here, try it out in your own life.

TAKE ADVANTAGE OF HEALTH CARE PROFESSIONALS IF YOU'RE HAVING TROUBLE GETTING STARTED

The most useful first step in goal setting is to look to others who know your situation for support. First and foremost is your own personal health care "team," including your neurologist, physical and occupational therapists, and others. These are people who you have grown to trust and who know you personally. Be sure to discuss any ideas you have for setting new goals for yourself with those who know you best, your health care team and your support partners.

SOME QUESTIONS TO PONDER

How many times have you set a goal, and never even started to follow through? In other words, how many times have you decided to lose weight, eat better, or get more exercise, and gotten nowhere? How many times has your goal been set, started up, and then gradually or suddenly given up? If you think about it, these are some of the very reasons why most of us tend to not keep our New Year's resolutions, and why most people over the age of 35 stop even bothering to make them!

The goals we set are difficult to achieve for a number of reasons. Very often, the goals we set are *too big*. Things like running the New York City Marathon next year or losing 100 pounds in 6 months are admirable but often larger than we can handle. Sometimes, the goals we set are *too complicated*. An example might be losing weight *and* getting a promotion at work *and* developing new relationships *and* improving our financial life. All of these goals, in and of themselves, are terrific, but taken together they can make us wonder if they can all be achieved. The goals we set are sometimes *too vague and not specific*. Statements like "working out more" or "feeling better about myself" are very difficult to get a handle on, not to mention the trouble we might have in measuring any real success.

2

Get the idea? Most of us set idealized goals in our lives even though we are unaware of the possibilities of attaining them. This is a universal human problem and one that can be approached in some very specific ways.

THE STAGES OF CHANGE

Most of us, at some time or another in our lives, reach a point when we know, deep down inside, that something in our lives has to change. Also, we realize that *we* have to be the ones to change it. There is a process to how we go about deciding to change—a process by which we can be effective at implementing change in our own lives. Basically, it involves five steps or stages that we all must go through during positive behavior change. This model is adapted from Prochaska and DiClemente. As you read through these stages, ask yourself:

- What stage of change you are in right now?

- Where you are in that process?

- What obstacles are standing in your way that might prevent you from reaching the next level, and ultimately success?

In doing this little exercise, you might want to have a particular goal in mind that is important to you. Go through each of these stages while staying aware of your current goal.

Stages of Change

1. *Pre-contemplation*—In this stage, a person is unaware that he or she really has a problem. There is no expressed desire to make any changes, and no real concern or immediacy for anything to be different. This is the "never" stage.
2. *Contemplation*—In this stage, a person has become aware that there may be a problem and has started to consider doing something about it. He or she may realize that his or her health could be in jeopardy and is beginning to "wish" that things could be different. This is the "someday" stage.

(continued)

Stages of Change (*continued*)

3. *Preparation*—When it is clear that the costs of maintaining your own behavior far outweigh the benefits, you may *decide* to do what it takes to change course. Here, we begin to think of every possible alternative and resource. This is the stage at which you develop your best plan to change your life's course and accomplish your goals. This is the "soon" stage.

4. *Action*—This is the stage in which you begin to implement your plan. You have prepared and feel physically, emotionally, and spiritually ready to embark on a journey to improve your life. This is the "now" stage.

5. *Maintenance*—This stage represents the phase where you begin to feel that you finally made it! You have successfully made the changes in your life that will lead you to your eventual goal. This is the "forever" stage. The danger of this final stage, after you've made some difficult changes, is that you might slide into complacency, begin to feel "bulletproof," and lose sight of some of the plans that were necessary to make this change.

SOURCES OF MOTIVATION

There are several different means by which people get motivated. Here is a short list:

■ *External motivation*
  This source of motivation comes completely from outside forces. For instance, if your health care provider told you to get more exercise or your support partner asked you to try to eat a healthier diet, you might well take that advice to heart and perhaps even start an exercise program or a new diet. Yet, if your sole source of motivation came from the urging of other people, studies show that the probability of your continuing this behavior is quite low. In other words, the goals that

you have set will probably not be permanent if your motivation is external. How much of your current motivation to change is external?

- *Identified motivation*
This source is based on the well-known "modeling effect." When people are exposed to new behaviors in friends, family, or individuals that they strive to be like, a process of modeling or imitation is likely to occur. If you have a friend who enjoys walking and you are invited to go along, you might find that you enjoy it more than if you were to do it alone. This also keeps you more accountable. Many people enjoy going to gyms and health clubs for this very reason. They see people who they want to be like and tend to identify with their behavior. As it turns out, this is a fairly strong source of motivation. You may simply want to be more like someone you identify with, making behavior change much easier.

- *Internal motivation*
When we internalize motivation, we tend to see our goals and plans as things we want to do for ourselves. People often comment, "This is for me," "I do it because it's a challenge," or "I like it because it's fun." You are in charge of your own life. If you want to make it happen, the next moves (and all the future moves) are up to you.

The P.A.U.S.E. Principle©

You can remember the acronym P.A.U.S.E. and use it as a motivational tool.

*P*lan your strategy
*A*ccount for changes
*U*nderstand your barriers
*S*low your pace
*E*xercise your options

GOALS VERSUS PLANS

One important point to consider here is the important difference between two words that are sometimes used interchangeably: goals and plans. A goal without a plan remains just a goal—many people have visions, intentions, ideas, and dreams that never happen because they are never planned.

- A **goal** is defined as the result or achievement *toward which effort is directed*. That is, a goal is the end result that one wishes to achieve. Goals often represent the "big picture" result of our efforts.

- **Goal setting** involves establishing *specific, measurable, and time-targeted objectives* to be achieved.

- A **plan** is defined as a scheme, program, or method worked out beforehand for the accomplishment of a goal or objective. In other words, it is the act of formulating a definite *course of action* or plan of attack.

SETTING A GOAL

As you think about your current situation right now, does any area stand out as needing attention? You might read through the titles of the other chapters in this book to give you ideas. Perhaps you might think of the area that has been the most difficult for you to change in the past, one where you have always struggled to keep yourself motivated and gotten stuck. This is the easy part. What is your goal today?

MAKING A PLAN

Some of the benefits of planning are:

- Planning *promotes focus*, since it is a disciplined thought process about your future.

- Planning *provides standards*, helping you to check your performance and measure your progress.

- Planning *prepares the planner*, so you are ready for any inevitable roadblocks or bumps in the road.

- Planning *stimulates thinking*, providing the stimulation needed to avoid dead ends and blind alleys.

- Planning *fuels confidence*, since it reduces the paralyzing effects of fear.

LARGE GOALS VERSES SMALL STEPS

Large goals alone, like New Year's resolutions, lead to anxiety and fear, and can ultimately lead to failure. Instead, think of taking small steps. The hardest thing to do when embarking on a new strategy, something you are trying to change, is to take the first step. Most tasks are 90 percent mental and 10 percent physical. That being said, if you work on taking small steps, it will help ease, if not eliminate, most of the fear and anxiety connected to big changes. It is clear how detrimental fear and anxiety are in our lives.

Think of a goal you've set in the past but did not complete. Maybe your last New Year's resolution! In many instances, our brains may not fully accept the large goals we set and we tend to turn away from them. The part of the brain called the amygdala is the area that generates fear and anxiety. When a large goal is set the amygdala becomes very active, and as a result the anxiety prevents us from ever attaining that goal. Plans, however, are your daily strategies to reach your goal. When we make a small plan, we basically trick our brains and bypass the fear reaction from the amygdala. Remember, the small, simple steps that you make each day can often turn into giant leaps!

Make a SMART Plan

Develop a SMART plan. Each letter describes an important component.

Specific/Simple: Plans should be straightforward and put an emphasis on what you want to happen. Being specific helps us to focus our efforts and clearly define what we are going to do. The specific part is the What and How of your SMART plan. *What* are you going to do? Be sure to use action words here. How are you going to do it? Be sure the plans you set are very specific, clear, and easy. Instead of making a goal to lose weight and be healthier, set a specific plan to walk in place for 10 minutes a day while watching the news.

(continued)

Make a SMART Plan (*continued*)

Measurable: If you can't measure it, you cannot manage it. Be sure to pick a plan with measurable progress, so you can see the changes occur. How will you know when you reach your goal? Be specific. The plan "I want to read 100 pages per day for the next six days" shows the specific target to be measured. "I want to be a better reader" is not measurable.

Attainable: As you identify the goal that is most important to you, you should begin to figure out ways that you can make that goal come true. As you develop these plans, make certain that the plans are actually things that you can accomplish and can imagine yourself doing.

Realistic: Realistic doesn't necessarily mean "easy." But in this case, realistic means something "do-able," and that the skills needed to do the work are available. Also, the project needs to fit with the overall strategy and goals. Try to devise a plan or a way of getting there which makes the goal realistic. For instance, a goal of "never again eating sugary foods" may not be realistic for someone who really enjoys and craves those foods. It might be more realistic to make a plan to eat one piece of fruit every day instead of a sugary sweet item. That way, you can choose to reduce the amount of sweets gradually in a plan that seems realistic to you.

Time-based: Be sure to set a time frame for the plan. A starting time is especially important, whether it is tomorrow morning at 10 o'clock, next Tuesday, or next month. Be sure the time frame that you choose is attainable and realistic for your life.

Remember, there is immense power in planning. This is what you expect to do each day.

Plans are your daily strategies to reach your goal, which are more easily accepted by your brain.

Formulate a SMART plan. Make a small, simple plan for change right now!

WHAT CAN I DO?

Make a small plan right now. First, restate your primary goal.

GOAL: _____

ACCOUNT FOR CHANGES

Many studies of behavior change indicate that when people keep track of the things they are trying to change, they tend to be more successful than if they don't monitor those changes. In fact, some research shows that the mere act of self-monitoring can often begin the process of behavior change. Despite these findings, most people flounder or fail at goal setting because they are not paying as much attention to daily changes as they should. They tend to be less mindful of small steps toward their goal.

Let's assume that a major area you want to change is your level of activity and exercise. A great example might be simply wearing a pedometer, just a simple one that counts steps taken each day. If you were to keep track of the number of steps you take every day, this would not only give you a baseline or starting point but you might also find that certain activities during your average day increase that number of steps.

The most important point here is to keep really good notes. Make sure you select things that are likely to change over time. Self-monitoring appears to make people more aware of small changes that they make every day.

It is important to remember that there are many methods of keeping track of changes or self-monitoring. Some people actually keep a daily journal in which they make regular entries. Still others might keep a behavior log, detailing the amount of time spent exercising during each day. This information can be collected on a daily calendar, something as simple as an index card or perhaps even on your computer or smart phone. Although there are many possible forms of self-monitoring, it is important for you to think about the format that would be most convenient for you. How will you keep track of progress?

WHAT CAN I DO?

Although you can be as creative as you wish, please select a means by which you will keep track of changes in your first simple plan. How will you account for your changes? What is your method for tracking progress?

UNDERSTAND YOUR BARRIERS

When trying to make a healthy behavior change, there will always be barriers in front of you, both before you start and along the way. The barriers being discussed are: external barriers, internal barriers, brain chatter, and time traps.

- *External barriers*
  These are barriers that occur naturally in all of our lives. External barriers might include major life changes that are largely out of our control. Some examples might be divorce, financial hardship, death of a loved one, or not having any training in strategic planning. Another external barrier might include disagreement with the goal setter, in which someone other than yourself has set a goal that you don't fully believe in and might not necessarily follow through with. Also, a significant external barrier is negative feedback from others. This occurs when you set out to follow through with your plan and others around you tell you that you probably won't succeed. For example, a spouse who discourages you from a new exercise plan since you have "never followed through with these plans in the past." Carefully examine your own life right now to see if any of these or other external barriers exist.

- *Internal barriers*
  These are barriers that we basically set up inside ourselves. The most frequent of these is based on the idea that you "can't teach an old dog new tricks." In other words, our own resistance to change because of the long-held belief that our behavior patterns have been established a long time ago and are unlikely to change. Another internal barrier to consider is psychological distress. It is well known

that many people with MS experience depression and anxiety. Untreated depression and anxiety can slow anyone down in getting the energy to complete new plans. Lastly, one of your internal barriers might simply be the fact that before today you had no plans. As we have seen in this chapter, careful plans are of utmost importance. Now look at your own internal barriers and see if they fit into these or any other categories.

■ *Brain chatter*

When we speak of "brain chatter," we are referring to all of the conversations that we have in our heads all day long. Many of these forms of brain chatter are examples of unhelpful thoughts. For instance, one unhelpful thought category is *rehashing the past*. Many people live in the past, especially if they have had some negative experiences that they can't get out of their minds. Some examples might be childhood abuse, a bitter divorce, or other sources of anger and resentment. How much of your time is spent rehashing the past?

Another type of brain chatter is *all-or-nothing thinking*. The basic idea behind this kind of chatter is exemplified by the phrase, "Either I do this perfectly or I will fail." This type of thinking requires that we see everything in terms of pure black-and-white, with no shades of gray. As you can imagine, this chatter will never allow us to feel as though we have partially succeeded, even if we attain 75 percent of our goal.

Yet another category of unhelpful chatter is called *disqualifying the positive*. Let's say you make your plans for the day and perform almost everything perfectly and on schedule. Despite this, you have one little slip in some area during that day. What is the one thing you will tend to remember? It's often that little slip. Our memories of our own successes and failures often reveal that we tend to dwell on our daily shortcomings and forget about those many things at which we have probably succeeded perfectly.

And finally, a kind of unhelpful thought that is the opposite of rehashing the past is one called *misfortune telling*. In this case, the focus is entirely on the future and on all the bad things that might lie ahead. Misfortune-telling chatter usually begins with the simple phrase, "What if?" Such as "What if my MS gets worse?" or "What if

I go bankrupt?" or "What if I get fired at work?" Misfortune-telling is all about anticipating future events, usually negative ones. How often do you wake up in the middle of the night and think, "Tomorrow will probably be a great day?" People have a tendency to look ahead, which of course is necessary for good planning, but very often we tend to look at many of the negative outcomes over which we have no control.

■ *Time traps*

Everyone has time traps. The most frequent excuse heard for not exercising is "I didn't have the time." Some people have very busy schedules and find it genuinely difficult to fit things in, even when they know they are good for them. Healthy eating and exercise are two of these. On the other hand, other people have a great deal of time in their day and still find it hard to accomplish their plans. Examine your own life right now and look at your daily schedule. How will you set up a plan to accomplish your goals? Whether you have a tight schedule each day or a fairly loose one, both ends of the spectrum can be time traps. What are your time traps?

WHAT CAN I DO?

As you read through the different kinds of barriers that you might encounter in accomplishing your plan, try to list the main categories that will make it difficult for you.

What are your external barriers?

_____

_____

What is a small step you could take to overcome any external barriers?

_____

What are your internal barriers?

_____

_____

What is a small step you could take to overcome any internal barriers?

_____

What types of brain chatter do you find yourself using?

_____

What is a small step you could take to overcome your brain chatter?
(e.g., learn mindfulness meditation; read a book on cognitive-behavior therapy)

_____

What are your time traps?

_____

_____

What is a small step you could take to overcome your time traps?
(e.g., make a daily schedule; use better time management)

_____

SLOW YOUR PACE

One of the most important parts of goal setting is taking some time out of each day to slow your pace. This is important for several reasons. First, the effects of stress on motivation are well known. Stress has a way of slowing us down in our present goals, since the orientation is usually toward the future and fears of what might happen. Your body needs a chance to recover during each day, and taking some time for stress management is just as important as sleeping and exercising properly.

Secondly, one of the known effects of stress is that it directs our minds to future fears and concerns, leaving no time for the present. Taking a bit of time each day to just be still and present with your body and mind will allow you a good avenue for considering those small and simple plans that you make each day.

Sometimes the signs of stress can be seen in the body, including tension in muscles, clenched teeth, or rapid shallow breathing. People with MS often have symptoms of fatigue and muscle tension, which might either be symptoms of the MS itself or stress. Knowing what causes or increases stress is often the first step in counteracting it. There are many great methods available that you might utilize to slow your pace.

One technique that is particularly useful in this setting is called mindfulness meditation. This is not only a great way to reduce "brain chatter" and calm the mind but it is also an excellent tool for increasing motivation and staying focused on the goal. The basic idea of mindfulness is very simple on the one hand, but subtle on the other. The only two ingredients necessary to be mindful of are (1) being physically still and (2) being mentally "present."

Here is one method for using mindfulness as a motivational tool. It is a great way to clear the clutter in your mind for a few minutes each day and stay on track.

Rule of 3 and 3

Every day, take 3 minutes some time in the morning, when you can be calm and quiet, to develop and visualize 3 simple plans—important but easy things that you can accomplish that day.

What can I do?_____

What can I do now to slow my pace?_____

EXERCISE YOUR OPTIONS

Now is the time to put it all together! In the previous exercises, you have been asked to

1. pick out a goal to focus on
2. develop a simple but specific plan or strategy
3. commit yourself to a way of keeping track of your progress
4. think through the barriers that you might encounter and possible ways to overcome them
5. explore ways to slow your pace during the day

DAMAGE CONTROL

Every person who tries to accomplish a goal will not perform at 100 percent efficiency. One of the scary questions that inevitably come up in our minds is, "What if I slip backwards?" You will inevitably have days like this, and this is exactly the time to use good damage control techniques. If you develop your plan through this material and start to act on it, you might well have a lapse along the way. This is the time to recommit yourself to your plans or even revise them in some way so that they fit the criteria we talked about earlier. Remember the power of affirmations, too. If you should have a lapse, say to yourself **"Tomorrow is another day,"** brush yourself off, and start over again. Another affirmation that is extremely powerful is the phrase from Alcoholics Anonymous, **"One day at a time."** You are certainly welcome to develop your own affirmation as well, and if you find a phrase that works for you, write it down on a yellow sticky and put it on your bathroom mirror!

Your Master Plan to Reach Your Goal ★

Goal _____

Plan _____

_____

On (date)_____ at (time) _____

I will _____

_____

(continued)

Your Master Plan to Reach Your Goal (*continued*)

I will keep track of my progress by _____

_____

I expect the following barriers _____

_____

I will overcome these barriers by _____

_____

I will slow my pace daily by (methods) _____

_____

REFERENCE

Prochaska, J. O., & DiClemente, C. C. (1998). Toward a comprehensive model of change. In W. R. Miller & N. Heather (Eds.) *Treating addictive behaviors: processes of change* (2nd Ed), p. 3-27. New York: Plenum Press.

2 Teamwork for a More Complete Health Care

Randall T. Schapiro

One of the most important and earliest decisions for you to make in managing your multiple sclerosis is forming a team of individuals who will be dedicated to maintaining your good health. This includes general health as well as neurological well-being. The health care team should be made up of a group of people you can be comfortable with and can trust to help manage your MS over time.

Typically, people see their providers on an as needed basis or as a regularly scheduled appointment. In the case of chronic illness, there are two main issues:

- The usual health and wellness visits may occur less often as more attention is given to multiple sclerosis.

- Chronic illnesses may require more intervention than what can be provided by a single provider.

Forming a health care team that includes general providers for overall health as well as MS specific providers will make the journey with MS easier. In addition to medical or rehabilitative team members, it is important to look to community activities, homes, the workplace, recreation activities, and resources for independent function. When forming the health care team, the person living with MS and his or her support partner should be the most important members and should be

MS Team

MS organizations

Financial advisor   Vocational counselor

Friends   Primary care provider

Support groups   Neurologist

Social worker   MS nurse

Psychologist/
Neuropsychologist   Community health

**Person with
MS**

Psychiatrist   Physical therapist

Physiatrist   Occupational
                     therapist
Urologist   Speech
             therapist

directing how needs are met. While forming this team may take time, health care teams enable whole health for the whole person.

In developing the "MS Team," attention to the merging of the personalities involved is essential. This will make up the "chemistry" of the interactions, and good chemistry will lead to more comfortable relationships. It takes time and thought to put together the proper composition of people, and the team members may change over time. The first thing to think about is the personality style of the person with MS. Is this individual a decision maker or someone who wants decisions made for them? Is this person assertive about his or her needs? These questions require honest answers without assessing value judgments.

In a similar manner, the various team members should be reviewed. In choosing the team members, the questions must be asked:

■   Is this person one who listens well and collaborates?

■   Is this person a team player or one who likes to go at it alone?

■   Is this person someone who will let the person with MS make all the decisions, without providing input?

Ideally, team members offer educated advice that is discussed and understood so that all are in agreement. In a similar manner the person living with MS may offer management suggestions that should be considered and implemented as appropriate. It is very important to respect the advice given by each member of the team while trying to find what is best for the health of the individual.

Medicine has come a long way in the past couple of decades. Evidence-based medicine is medical advice based on studies that have shown that something works (efficacy). In addition, it is appropriate to add treatments that have not necessarily been studied as vigorously but are effective. That may be called "complementary" medicine and include such things as nutritional supplements, types of exercise and therapy, some psychological and meditation techniques, and so on. In either case, health care providers should be able to offer opinions on treatment options and patients should be able, after listening to the options, to make their own treatment choices.

WHAT CAN I DO?

Establish care with a primary care provider to attend to total health for the whole you.

Understand your personal style regarding health care so you can choose the providers who best match your style.

THE PLAYERS

Finding the right neurologist is central to ongoing MS management. Asking others in the community their experiences regarding physicians may be helpful. The National MS Society has a list of interested and qualified physicians. Sometimes the health plans of an individual dictate the care. It may be necessary to travel a distance to find the necessary relationship. There is nothing wrong with doing that; the visits are not likely to be frequent but are very important.

Finding a primary health care provider to manage the non-MS health issues is equally important, and that person's office should be closer in location. It is helpful for the neurologist and the primary health provider to have a communication plan such as phone calls, electronic records, e-mails, or an exchange of letters. The person with MS may have to actually set this up for it to work efficiently, and remind the professionals to correspond in some fashion periodically. Having MS does not prevent other diseases from occurring, so the relationship between the neurologist and primary health care provider is essential.

MS can be a lonely disease, but it should not be. The support of others is extremely important. Thus, when forming the health team, a support partner (a friend, a spouse or a relative) is an important addition. Determining that person and his or her role is invaluable.

The other members of the health care team are variable. All people with MS may not need every member of the team but some may. Being open to the concept of a health care team allows the team to grow. Here are some examples of team members:

- Physiatrists are physicians who specialize in rehabilitation and physical medicine. They work closely with the rehabilitation therapists and neurologists in coordinating patient care and sometimes will serve as the team leader.

- Nurse practitioners (NP) are nurses who have completed course and experience work beyond that of basic nursing and are called "advanced practice nurses." They may prescribe medication and function in many ways as a physician might.

- Registered nurses (RN) have completed education and course work to be licensed by the state as educationally proficient to help patients at a high nursing level.

- Licensed practical (vocational) nurses (LPN) have less formal education than the registered nurse but often have vast practical experience accompanying their education and can be very helpful in teaching and managing issues of patients.

- Physician assistants (PA) have advanced educational preparation to help physicians manage medical problems. They may prescribe medications and function as a physician would.

- Medical assistants have been taught to assist in the office with multiple issues that arise.

- Physical therapists (PT) have gone to a university to study the mechanics of the human body in health and disease. Depending on their education and interest they may emphasize orthopedic/sport issues and/or neurological problems. In MS the neurological therapist is involved in teaching people how to maximize function depending on abilities or disabilities. This involves assessment of the symptoms a person has and establishing a treatment program to address those symptoms. They also can recommend assistive devices and train people in their use.

■ Occupational therapists (OT) work at the "occupation" of living. They teach people how to do the activities of daily living efficiently. This may include dressing, eating, bathing, grooming, toileting, household chores, and workplace demands. Some have more experience with visual problems and some are skilled in working with cognitive problems.

■ The speech/language pathologist (SLP) may be involved in speech therapy involving voice and speech but they also play an important role in swallowing as well as evaluating and managing cognitive problems.

■ The nutritionist or registered dietician (RD) is educated to teach people how to make healthy dietary choices.

■ Psychiatrists are physicians who focus on mental health issues and can prescribe psychological medications. They often just manage medications and recommend other professionals for talk therapy.

■ Clinical psychologists primarily focus on individual and group counseling. Psychologists also work with families.

■ Some social workers have taken educational course work to become licensed to be Mental Health professionals providing counseling for individuals and groups.

■ Neuropsychologists primarily focus on doing neuropsychological testing, analyzing the findings, and directing future care to address those findings.

■ The social worker may be involved in managing the community services and benefits and placement of people into positions of success. They may not be constant members of the team but may be necessary from time to time.

■ Support groups are available in many communities. They may be professionally led or peer led. Groups can offer needed support and education but each group is different and not everyone enjoys group experiences.

■ Financial advisors can offer advice for anyone at any stage in life. Having MS may prompt a person to seek advice for the future early in the diagnosis and not to wait until later in the disease.

■ MS organizations such as the National MS Society, the Multiple Sclerosis Association of America, the Multiple Sclerosis Foundation, Can Do MS, and the Consortium of MS Centers are resources for:
   • Information, education
   • Services
   • Support groups
   • Newsletters and calendars of events
   • Social support
   • Referral services
   • Public programs, social opportunities, and recreational activities

It is beneficial to understand who may be involved on the health care team before stresses occur. In fact, the stresses may never occur, but to feel secure is important.

WHAT CAN I DO?

Set up your health care team based on your provider's recommendations, advice from MS organizations, or discussion with other people living with MS.

MS CENTERS

In the past two decades "comprehensive" MS Centers have appeared on the scene. These centers often have the team already formed, either within their walls or in the geographical area. Communication is the key to good team practice. It matters little whether the physical therapist is down the hall or down the block if there is appropriate communication of needs back and forth. Many communities do not have the luxury of a comprehensive center and the team has to be put together individually.

Team formation outside of MS Centers can be stressful for both patients and providers as they develop communication styles and come to understand each other's needs. It is doable, but clearly more difficult. Managed care insurance plans often play a role in what services may be covered, by whom they may be provided, and how often one can receive them. Learning how insurance plans work and what benefits are covered is crucial for good care.

COMMUNICATION

There are various ways communication between team members can take place: in person, by telephone, and exchanging medical records or e-mail. It may be smooth and coordinated or less so, but what is important is that communication takes place. There needs to be clear instructions as to who is responsible for what. Much of this involves short term intervention, but some of it may require long term planning.

With a good team in place, many of the stresses and insecurities of the unknown may vanish. Living with multiple sclerosis becomes far more comfortable. The providers need to know the potential referral resources, and the person with MS should feel confidence in the professionalism of the team.

INSURANCE ISSUES

In today's world, the insurance company may feel they have the final word in the members of the team by using reimbursement as the decision maker. From that perspective, the team members may be determined by who is participating in the insurance plan's choice of participating professionals. The insurance company may provide a case manager or care manager. That can be a distinct advantage if that individual has MS quality management as the goal. However, if he or she is a manager of costs, there may be debate over needed services. Patients are encouraged to be their own advocates whenever possible. If provider and patient agree that an evaluation, medication, or use of an adaptive aid is needed, and the request is denied, it often becomes the role of the patient to follow through. Asking for help from the provider will probably be necessary, but patient persistence will be needed. Utilization of community resources will be needed as well.

THE APPOINTMENT

At each appointment with any team member, care and time should be taken, by the person living with MS or their support partner, to have a list of questions. Answers should be noted and potentially written to ensure that they are remembered. Questions regarding research and clinical trials may be brought up. A person with MS should be interested in evidence-based medicine, but may have questions about other strategies available to help certain symptoms and situations. Questions should be prioritized with the most important at the top, since appointment times may be limited and not allow adequate time for all questions. Time is of the essence, and efficient utilization of time is necessary.

WHAT CAN I DO?

- Have a list of questions
- Record answers
- Ask questions about new research
- Talk about symptoms
- Prioritize questions knowing you may not get them all asked

Team forming is an essential beginning to the journey with MS and should occupy a significant amount of time and thought. A good start may well determine a more successful course of management and an improved quality of life.

3 Living With the Challenge

Peggy Crawford

There are several things about MS that make it challenging. Once MS is on the scene, it makes its presence known on most if not all days. Living with MS is like living with an uninvited guest that never goes home and leaves clutter all over the house. MS is unpredictable. Symptoms can change from hour to hour and day to day. Activities that can be done on Monday might not be possible by Wednesday. New symptoms start and old symptoms can come back. Exacerbations can leave behind symptoms that act as a reminder that MS is here to stay. MS takes up lots of time, energy, and money. Living with MS involves making decisions about treatment, disclosure, employment, relationships, and plans for the future. MS is commonly associated with losses in function and roles, resulting in changes for people with MS and the people in their lives. For example, having to give up the role of family breadwinner, the person who has always been responsible for the outside work at home, or the parent who has primarily taken care of the children, are experienced as significant losses. Such losses are likely to be associated with feelings of grief.

Grief is a normal and universal reaction to loss. Although many people associate grief only with death, loss can be experienced when a chronic illness is diagnosed. Beyond diagnosis, grief can be experienced periodically as additional losses occur with changes in the illness. This is commonly the case with MS. Grief can include feelings of sadness, anger, and fear, as well as yearnings for whatever people thought their life would have been without MS. Even in the early phase of MS, people can experience the loss of what their life was like before MS. They can experience the loss of self, identity, independence, and control even when their symptoms are invisible to others. Grief can occur at any time, even when function has not changed. People grieve what they feel they have already lost and what they anticipate could be lost, including relationships, job, health insurance, and retirement.

If skills and abilities change, grief is likely to occur again. In MS, an important part of grief is reviewing what used to be. For example, some people who are no longer able to walk are still walking in their dreams. It's important to remember that grief does not mean that someone has given up. Grief is normal. It is not the same as depression and does not necessarily require treatment with medication. Having the opportunity to talk with someone about the feelings experienced with grief can be helpful. There is no schedule or time limit on grieving. It is experienced differently by each individual, and like so many things in MS, one size does not fit everyone.

Information in this chapter applies to people with MS and the people in their lives, especially support partners. As you read this consider these questions:

1. How do I usually deal with stressful situations and problems in my life?
2. Do I think about MS as a threat, a challenge, or both?
3. What do I find most challenging about living with MS?
4. What can I do to be a healthy person with MS in my life?
5. What coping skills do I already have and what new skills or tools do I need?

Coping is a process that includes what people think, feel, and do in stressful situations. Sometimes people are not aware of what they think and feel when stressed, but they usually know what they do. Steps in the coping process include defining the problem, generating possible solutions, trying out solutions, evaluating how well the solution worked, and trying another solution if the situation does not seem better. Effective coping can help to reduce stress and emotional distress.

For most people, learning how to cope effectively is a lifelong process. It can help to think of effective coping as a toolbox that is always available and ready for use whenever it's needed. Effective coping requires lots of practice with different tools for different situations and keeping those tools in good working order. As life changes, new tools can be added and old tools can be removed. Over time, tools can become rusty from lack of use. Sometimes, they can just be dusted off, have that rust removed, and be sharpened for use. Other times, tools that do not work need to be removed or at least put aside for a while. It's important to try and keep the toolbox balanced. For example, a toolbox containing five hammers and no screwdriver or wrench would not be very useful. Remember, MS is likely to present with a variety of challenges, and not all tools work for all challenges. In MS, a combination of these tools is likely to result in an improved quality of life:

■ Close friends and family

■ Healthy habits (good sleep, diet, and exercise)

■ Engaging in relaxing and distracting activities

■ Effective problem-solving skills

■ Having a purpose in life

THINKING OF MS AS A THREAT OR A CHALLENGE

It is common for people with MS to experience their MS diagnosis and the changes that come with it as threatening or challenging. When people think of their MS as a threat, they are usually waiting for the other shoe to drop, walking around as if there is a black cloud looming over their shoulder, and focusing on the unpredictability of their condition. They tend to experience MS as overwhelming. This can be anxiety-provoking and scary. People who think of MS in this way are sometimes afraid to move (literally and otherwise) or make plans because something might go wrong. They decide to not take a new job, move into a 2-story house, or return to school as they dreamed about doing, because they don't know what the future holds. They do not go on the family cruise that was planned a year ago and looked forward to by everyone because they do not want to be away from home and their doctor "just in case." They do not go on the outing to the zoo because there's too much walking around and they do not want to be seen walking with any assistive device such as a cane or rollator. As a result, they miss out on lots of activities that would likely be fun and a chance to spend time with people they love and who love them. Life can start to feel like it is standing still. Sometimes, people are so focused on what might go wrong in the future, they miss what is going on in the present. They feel surrounded by MS and controlled by it rather than feeling like they have any control. They can become immobilized by MS even when able to walk. They often live in the past and dread the future because it is unknown. They can get stuck in asking "why me?" and wanting "my old life back."

When people think of their MS as a challenge, it can be an opportunity to step back and examine how things have been done until now and come up with ways of doing things differently. For example, people may focus on better conservation of energy to reduce fatigue and improve quality of life for themselves and their family. Learning how to deal with the challenges in life is an ongoing process with limitless opportunities to make changes and try new things. Many people with MS find that the diagnosis motivates them to live a healthier life and make changes they have been meaning to make for years. They consider both their physical and emotional health. They start to exercise, eat better, and get more sleep. They manage their fatigue more effectively by not overdoing, and avoid being exhausted for days. They take more time for important relationships with family and friends. They think about the primary sources of stress, eliminate those they can, and come up with healthier ways of dealing with those they can't. MS can provide the opportunity to think outside the box, be creative, and add new tools to that box. These people plan for the future but live in the present.

Many people with MS experience it as both a threat and a challenge. When an exacerbation occurs or a big decision needs to be made, it can feel pretty threatening, but it's also a challenge. If MS is mostly thought of as a challenge, it sits beside you so you can look at it if you want to, reach out and touch it when you need to, but it's not in front of you as an obstacle that will keep you from moving forward. When seen as a challenge, people will try something even when the outcome isn't known because they have a backup plan, sort of like the cane that's kept in the car just in case. Given the choice, it's better to go with the cane in the car rather than stay home and miss out.

There is no doubt that life with MS can feel like a test or moving into unchartered waters. For many people diagnosed with MS, they have never been seriously ill before. They may not have seen a doctor regularly or taken prescription medication regularly. The reality is that healthy people get MS. For most people with MS the challenges start early and continue throughout life. Although some challenges occur only at the time of diagnosis, other challenges, such as decisions about treatment, come up periodically and are not necessarily related to how long someone has had MS.

Challenges to Be Discussed

- Diagnosis
- Starting treatment
- Interactions with the health care system
- Disclosing information about MS
- Changes in functions, roles, and responsibilities
- Changes in relationships with family, friends, and coworkers
- MS-related decisions and transitions
- Invisible symptoms

DIAGNOSIS

As many people know, getting diagnosed can be a challenge all by itself. People can have nonspecific symptoms for years that don't immediately point to MS. Also, symptoms can come and then disappear just as someone is thinking about going back to the doctor. Many of the symptoms are invisible. Getting to the right doctor can be challenging. People can be told they have something other than MS. Dealing with insurance companies can be frustrating and take lots of time.

When the diagnosis is made, people react in different ways. Some people feel shocked and think, "This can't be happening to me, I've always been a healthy person." Others quickly move into denial and think, "Maybe this will go away or they made the wrong diagnosis." It is normal to experience a combination of feelings. Many people feel anxious, wondering, "What does this mean for my future?"; angry because "This isn't fair"; and guilty because "I'm letting my family down," all at the same time. It is not unusual for people to feel relieved that they have an explanation for their symptoms and know that treatments are available while also feeling sad and angry that it is not something that can be cured.

STARTING TREATMENT

After the diagnosis is made, decisions about treatment need to be considered. There are several treatments available, but having several choices can make the decision feel overwhelming. It can be helpful for the person with MS to realize that they are not alone in making this decision. It is also helpful to think about how she or he wants to go about making this decision. Many people with MS want a team to help them with this process. One thing to think about is who will be on this team and what is expected of each person. Some people prefer that the physician make the final decision based on what is known about the person's test results, symptoms, and condition. Others want the physician to make a recommendation but want to make the final decision together with their support person. Most people want information about the different treatment options, especially how often the medication has to be taken and the possible side effects. Not everyone goes about this in the same way. Some people want to read educational materials about the different medications while others prefer to watch the video. Some people talk with other people who have MS to find out what they take. People want to choose a medication that will work well, cause the least side effects, and fit with their lifestyle.

Sometimes, support partners and family members have strong opinions about the course of treatment the person with MS should follow. It is not unusual for these opinions to not match up to those of the person who actually has MS. For example, if the symptoms seem mild and are not interfering with everyday life, including work, one person might want to take a wait and see approach while the other person may not want to wait because of what could happen without treatment. Sometimes one person is anxious for treatment to be started while the other person is worried about side effects and whether treatment is even necessary. Some people are very concerned about the cost of treatment and how much their health insurance will cover. These differences of opinion and worries can add to the stress of the MS diagnosis. Talking about the options and starting treatment is the beginning of a lifelong process of trying to balance the costs and benefits when making decisions about MS. These decisions are complicated because there is a lot of information to digest, several options to consider, and the decisions affect the lives of multiple people, including the person with MS and the people who support them.

INTERACTIONS WITH THE HEALTH CARE SYSTEM

It doesn't take long for people to realize that MS symptoms vary a lot and are unpredictable: "Here today, gone tomorrow, and back in a week." Exacerbations are likely to present different coping challenges than day-to-day symptoms. Exacerbations may require significant changes that are often temporary, while day-to-day symptoms are likely to require changes and adjustments that can vary in amount and degree but are pretty much in place every day. Also, many symptoms are not visible to other people and are hard to describe. In spite of being invisible, symptoms can still affect what people with MS are able to do. Talk about challenging!

Deciding when to call the provider also can be challenging. People with MS often ask themselves:

- What symptoms or changes in symptoms should be reported?

- How long should I wait to call?

- Does it have to be a new symptom or an old symptom that has gotten worse?

- What if I can still do most of what I need to do but it's much harder?

- What counts as an exacerbation? How do I know when it is my MS or something else?

Many people with MS are concerned about how their doctor and the office staff will react to their calls. For example, "Will they think I'm exaggerating my symptoms or overly concerned? I know they're busy people and I'm taking up their valuable time. Maybe there's nothing that can be done and I just have to live with it. Maybe this is as good as it gets with MS."

It can be helpful to ask for specific guidelines (preferably in writing) that explain when to call the provider and what to call about. This is a good topic to bring up during one of the first visits after diagnosis because it can help people to feel more prepared when symptoms change. Asking questions about office procedures is also useful. For example, people often want to know who is likely to call them back, how long it usually takes for calls to be returned, and what additional information they should provide when they call. It is also important to know what to do when the office is closed. All of these strategies and tools can help to reduce the stress and challenges associated with the MS experience.

Navigating the insurance and health care systems is another challenge for people and families with MS. Many people have not interacted much with their insurance company or given much thought to their coverage. It can take months to schedule an appointment with a specialist such as a neurologist, and some specialists are not covered by certain plans. MS medications are expensive, and the medication prescribed may not be the one covered at the highest rate by a specific plan. Before MS, people often chose the least expensive plan with a high deductible because they did not expect to use their coverage very often. MS forces people to deal with their insurance company. Trying to make sense out of insurance coverage with copays and coinsurance payments can quickly feel overwhelming.

DISCLOSING INFORMATION ABOUT MS

Disclosing information about MS can be a particularly challenging decision. It is not always easy to decide who, what, when, or even whether to tell. This can feel like risky business because people's reactions to this news are not always predictable or helpful. Does this sound familiar? In a way, this experience is similar to MS symptoms that can vary so much. Disclosing MS opens the door for people to share their opinions and advice about MS even when they have little or no experience. They may make observations about whether or not the person with MS fits their idea of someone with MS, suggest treatments they have heard about, and give advice about employment and disability. Although these comments may be well intended, they can feel intrusive and hurtful at times. As people say, "You can't unring a bell," so people are encouraged to be selective when disclosing information about their MS.

Before disclosing, and when time allows, it can be helpful to think about the reasons for telling. What does the person with MS and his or her support person want to accomplish by talking about MS? For some people living with MS, they disclose because they want, need, and deserve support. They want someone to talk to about their MS and how it's affecting their life. In other circumstances, telling others the reason their walk looks different can be better than having others making assumptions that are often wrong and potentially harmful. Disclosure is another area where the person with MS and people in their support system might not agree about what to do. In an effort to support each other, it can be helpful to discuss this early on and come to some agreement about whom to share with and what will be shared in an effort to support each other. This decision can always be changed to include more people and information as MS changes. For example, some people choose to not tell elderly parents who are ill themselves, especially if they live at a distance and don't see them regularly. Others choose to not tell adult children until they come home to visit.

For some people, decisions about disclosure are affected by the type and severity of their symptoms. If people have mostly invisible symptoms, they might take more time to make these decisions. Other symptoms, such as difficulty walking, are more obvious so some disclosure is likely to occur earlier. Few people know much about the disease so it can be helpful for people and families with MS to prepare for the unexpected. For example, it's not unusual for people to say something like, "But you look so good, maybe they made the wrong diagnosis." It's not unheard of for people to ask, "Why aren't you in a wheelchair?" or describe the worst case scenario about the one person they knew with MS. Although talking about MS can be challenging, not talking about it doesn't always work very well. Keeping secrets can be stressful for the person with MS and their support partner. Keeping track of who knows and who doesn't is challenging. Not disclosing to anyone reduces opportunities to access the support needed by everyone involved.

At work and out in the community, disclosure paves the way for asking for help and using assistive devices if they're needed. Disclosure allows people to remain involved in activities and relationships that might otherwise be avoided. Remember, it's okay to pick and choose when disclosing about MS. Disclosure is a personal decision and the whole world doesn't need to know, but it usually works better to provide people with specific information about symptoms and how they affect day-to-day functioning rather than a label (e.g., most people won't know what Relapsing Remitting MS is). Information can be tailored to the person who is being told. For example, concrete information is better for younger children but school-aged children and teens can understand more complicated information and sometimes want to read about MS on their own. Offering people written information about MS can be helpful but not everyone will want to read it, so don't take it personally.

Disclosure at work is a particularly challenging issue. Sometimes, the person with MS decides that it's better for people at work to know why they are having difficulty walking or need to use a handicapped parking place rather than having those people make faulty assumptions. Sometimes a person will choose to not reveal their diagnosis. They might anticipate a negative response from coworkers or management. If a person with MS is able to do the job, they do not have to tell anyone in the workplace. The reality is that in some situations, knowledge of this diagnosis by others may have a negative effect for the person with MS; however, remember that most people know little or nothing about MS so there is an opportunity to provide accurate information. There are times when coworkers or supervisors make assumptions about what a person with MS is able to do. For example, they might decide that the person with MS is no longer able to do their job. A supervisor might even reduce job responsibilities without checking this out. As a result, many people with MS are proactive and disclose their diagnosis when their symptoms interfere with their job performance so they can take an active role in making changes or implementing accommodations that will help them stay on the job. When at least some coworkers know about the MS, it can provide much needed support. When disclosure is not made, it is not possible to ask for accommodations.

CHANGES IN FUNCTIONS, ROLES, AND RESPONSIBILITIES

Over time, most people with MS experience changes in how they function at home and at work. These changes are the result of MS symptoms that affect what a person is able to do, how fast they can do it, and how much they can do. When changes occur during an exacerbation they might be temporary, but in many cases changes occur more slowly over a number of years and stick around. It isn't always easy to know right away what is temporary and what is here to stay. When symptoms come and stay, they can challenge a person's ability to continue with their usual roles and responsibilities at home and at work. For example, if the person with MS has been responsible for yard work and repairs on the house but now has extreme fatigue, difficulty walking, and/or balance problems, these activities will be more difficult, fatiguing, and maybe even unsafe to do. This situation requires pretty much everyone in the situation to make some changes, such as taking on new responsibilities, trading jobs, and doing things together that were previously done independently

Sometimes the person with MS has been the primary breadwinner and the support partner stayed home with the children, but with increasing MS symptoms this might not be possible. In other circumstances, the person with MS has been the go-to person for the children but is no longer able to drive them to after-school activities. These changes in function that commonly occur in MS are often experienced as losses for the person with MS as well as the important people in their lives. Roles and responsibilities are part of a person's identity, and giving them up or doing them differently can feel like not being the same person. These changes and losses are some of the most challenging aspects of living with MS. Coming up with ways to maintain identity and self-esteem can be hard work, and this work is likely to come up more than once with MS.

CHANGES IN RELATIONSHIPS

With these changes in functions and roles come changes in relationships. This includes relationships with support partners, children, extended family, friends, and coworkers. For example, maybe the person with MS was always the person to manage the finances but now has trouble keeping the checkbook balanced and remembering to pay bills. Giving up this responsibility to another person is difficult, but so is taking on this responsibility—particularly if it's being added to an already long list. It's not surprising that increased tension and conflict occur for couples in this situation. These are difficult adjustments even for couples who have been in committed relationships for years before MS. As people take on new responsibilities and work together to get things done, good communication is one of the most important tools for the family toolbox.

For people who are not involved in a committed relationship at the time of diagnosis, the idea of starting a new relationship can be scary and overwhelming. In fact, it's not unusual for people to think, "Now I'm damaged goods, so who would want me? No one will want to take the chance of being with someone who might end up in a wheelchair. I don't want to be a burden to anyone." In spite of these concerns, people usually venture into the unpredictable world of relationships. In these circumstances, the issue of disclosure looms large. When MS symptoms are visible, disclosure usually comes earlier in the relationship. When symptoms are invisible, people often spend more time thinking about when and what to tell about their MS. People want to be honest but worry about scaring off potential partners. In general, if a relationship feels like it's worth pursuing, it's worth taking the risk and talking about MS.

Keep in mind that people don't need to hear everything at once. Too much information can be overwhelming to a potential support partner. Most people need time to digest information and ask questions before moving on. It's useful to find out if the person knows anything about MS or has ever known anyone with MS. When talking about MS symptoms, it's helpful to be specific about how symptoms are likely to affect shared activities and ways to manage symptoms so that joint interests can be pursued. For example, if both people enjoy out-of-doors activities but temperature sensitivity is an issue, activities can occur early or later in the day. It can also be helpful to offer information about MS or point people in the direction of resources such as the National MS Society and Can Do MS. Answering questions as they come up and checking in periodically with the person to see if they have questions is a good idea. In general, people will take their lead from the person with MS. If that person seems open to talking about MS, others are likely to feel more comfortable bringing it up.

MAKING MS-RELATED DECISIONS AND TRANSITIONS

Some decisions related to MS are likely to come up every day, such as how to use available energy, while other decisions, like whether or not go to the zoo with the family in the middle of summer, will come up periodically. There are likely to be decisions about the management and treatment of symptoms such as medications, PT and OT, and assistive equipment. There could also be decisions about working or driving that are major and life changing. These decisions affect the person with MS and the people in their support network. Sometimes there is a fair amount of time to make these decisions and sometimes they need to be made more quickly. Even in the early years of the disease, it's a good idea to gather information about insurance benefits, long term disability insurance, and financial planning that might be useful in the future.

INVISIBLE SYMPTOMS

There are often unique challenges related to invisible symptoms that include fatigue, pain, sensory changes (like numbness and tingling), vision problems, bladder and bowel problems, depression, and cognitive changes. Unlike some MS symptoms such as difficulty walking, that are obvious to other people, invisible symptoms cannot be seen, observed, or experienced by others. Sometimes it's hard to come up with a good description of the symptom that others can understand. It's not unusual for others to get a strange look on their face when a person with MS describes sensory symptoms such as, "It feels like something crawling under my skin." People tend to minimize what they can't see. Support partners and friends might say something like, "I get tired too, and it's normal to forget things." This can be frustrating to the person with MS because invisible symptoms can affect day-to-day functioning and get in the way just as much as visible symptoms. It can be particularly frustrating when support partners don't take the symptoms seriously or misinterpret them.

Let's use fatigue as an example. It's the most common symptom in MS. Fatigue can interfere with just about everything and is one of the primary reasons that people with MS leave the workforce early. There are many good descriptions of MS-related fatigue, including "small things feel heavy," "getting ready for work is work," "I have an overwhelming need to sleep," and "I crash and hit the wall." Fatigue can interfere with physical, mental, and social activities as well as mood. Support partners often think they "get it," in many cases because they really want to understand, but it's almost impossible for them to "get it" because it's not the same tiredness they experience. MS-related fatigue can be misinterpreted in many ways. Support partners and others have been known to conclude that fatigue is related to depression, lack of sleep, medication side effects, not enough exercise, and lack of effort or laziness. Even if well intended, these comments can feel hurtful and blaming. As a result, the person with MS might conclude that they have caused their own fatigue. At other times, the person with MS can unknowingly add to their fatigue by trying to live like they don't have MS. They might not ask for or accept help when it's offered. They might be inflexible about how they do things and believe that changing how they do things is equal to giving up and giving in to MS. Remember, it's about adjustment and balance!

INTERPERSONAL CHALLENGES

MS affects relationships with family, friends, and coworkers. People react in many ways to the news that someone has MS. They may even question the diagnosis. People have been known to make comments like: "Maybe they made a mistake"; "Maybe you should get another opinion"; "I thought people with MS were in a wheelchair." These comments can be particularly frustrating for someone who has spent months and sometimes years seeing health care professionals and going through testing. After an MS diagnosis, it is not unusual for people to freely provide "well-meant" advice including their recommendations for treatments. It can be a challenge just deciding how to respond to these people. Sometimes people want the person with MS to talk to another person they know with MS even though these two people might have little in common except for their MS. An appropriate response usually includes an expression of appreciation for the information and acknowledgment of their concern.

Personal relationships are likely to be affected by MS as well. For people who are already in a committed relationship, the support partner is likely to have knowledge of the symptoms, the testing, and the diagnosis, but this doesn't necessarily make it easier. Sometimes, people with MS worry that their support partner will not be able to handle the MS and will leave. People are often hesitant to talk about their fears but it's important to get them out in the open. In this way, good communication can be a useful tool right from the beginning.

COPING STYLES

Coping style refers to how people deal with stressful situations, and MS is a stressful situation. Not all people with MS or support partners cope with MS in the same way. Frequently used coping styles include unhealthy denial, over identification with MS, and healthy denial.

When people use "unhealthy" denial, (Figure 1) they seem to stay stuck in "why me" thinking no matter how long they've had MS. They might avoid traditional MS treatments or use them irregularly. For example, they might take their injections less frequently than prescribed because they're not sure the medication is working or they've never been convinced they needed it in the first place. They are likely to try unproven therapies. They are reluctant to use assistive equipment in spite of clear need. The person who won't use a cane "because of how it might look," but uses up valuable energy trying to stay upright and falls regularly is one example. They may be resistant to educating themselves about MS and believe that "it's all bad news and nothing will help." As a result, they can miss out on exciting news about treatments and resources for people with MS. They are less likely to become involved in MS support groups because they assume "it will be depressing" rather than providing the inspiration and encouragement that many people experience. They are like the ostrich with its "head in the sand" in this case: "If I don't think about MS, it isn't there."

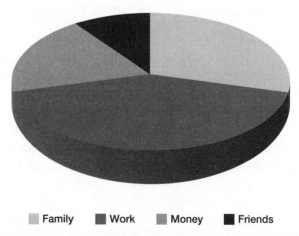

▪ Family   ▪ Work   ▪ Money   ▪ Friends

Figure 1 Unhealthy denial: MS isn't even on the radar

Others with MS become "over-identified" with their condition (Figure 2). They give up most if not all of their previous activities and friends. They spend much of their time thinking about and talking about MS by participating in support groups, on-line groups, and MS-related activities. They tend to think of themselves as disabled from early on in their MS experience. They tend to focus on what they can't do rather than what they can. Their identity is mostly about being a person with MS rather than a spouse, a worker, a parent, or a friend. They tend to separate themselves from family and friends and lose those important connections. Their life is really out of balance.

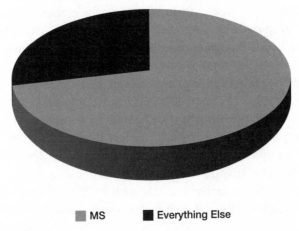

■ MS   ■ Everything Else

Figure 2 Over-identification with MS: It's taking up way too much space

On the other hand, people who use "healthy" denial maintain balance between MS and the rest of their life (Figure 3). They continue to carry out roles and responsibilities that they had before MS, even if they have to do them differently. They are flexible about how they do things. They ask for and accept help from others. They remain engaged with family and friends in activities and events. They are actively involved in the treatment of their MS, using a combination of prescribed medications and other strategies for managing symptoms. They are open to recommendations from the health care team, such as their PT and OT for rehab services, counseling services, and support groups as needed. When they talk about themselves, MS is not the first thing they mention. They view MS primarily as a series of challenges but realize that it will likely feel like a threat at times. They know that MS will always be part of their lives but those non-MS aspects of their identity remain in place.

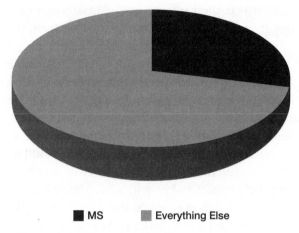

■ MS   ▨ Everything Else

Figure 3 Healthy denial: Life has some balance

People with healthy coping skills see MS as an opportunity for change and growth. They often re-evaluate their life and their priorities. For example, many people decide that more time with family and friends is a better investment than more time at the office. They look at their relationships and decide to spend less time with a friend who is always negative and more time with a friend who leaves them laughing. They look at their relationship with their support partner and work on improving communication and intimacy. In many cases, they consider MS to be the "kick in the butt" they needed to finally start living a healthier life. They start exercising, eating better, and losing weight. They look at how they handle stress, eliminate the stressors they can, and practice healthier ways of dealing with the many stressors that remain.

EXAMPLE OF EFFECTIVE COPING

Over time, many people with MS experience progression in their symptoms so that day-to-day functioning is affected and coping is challenged. Take walking as an example. Many people with MS have difficulty walking safely without some form of assistance such as a cane, rollator, or wheelchair. Unfortunately, many people are reluctant to use one of these devices because they anticipate embarrassment or feel that to do so indicates that they have given up. For some people, the use of an assistive device negatively affects their self-image and makes them feel dependent. As a result, they prefer to walk holding onto walls, furniture, or the arm of a support partner, which can result in more dependency. On the other hand, walking unsafely and falling can also result in unwanted attention. People with MS who cope more successfully in this situation are likely to think about the benefits and the costs of using and not using an assistive device. Benefits might include fewer falls and injuries, fewer misinterpretations of their walking, better fatigue management, and continued involvement in activities they enjoy. These activities could include attending their children's athletic and school events or staying in a job that helps to support their family and provides health insurance. Realistically, there are likely to be some costs such as the cost of the equipment, inconvenience, and maybe even some initial embarrassment. In spite of these costs, people who cope effectively are more likely to focus on achieving their goal even if this means doing something differently.

 Factors Associated With Effective Coping

- Positive attitude
- Social support
- Learning about MS
- Effective communication skills
- Effective stress management
- Asking for help and accepting help
- Dealing with emotional distress rather than ignoring it
- Problem-solving
- Flexibility
- Realistic goal setting
- Courage
- Seeking professional help as needed

Positive attitude—How people look at life seems to make a difference. Pessimists tend to see the glass as half empty, while optimists see the glass as half full. Having an optimistic attitude seems to be helpful when it comes to coping with the challenges of MS and in life in general. In addition, optimists are easier people to live with.

Social support—People are a valuable resource. They encourage the person with MS to keep trying, provide support when difficult decisions need to be made, come through when needed, are honest but gentle when giving feedback, and can disagree while showing respect.

Learning about MS—Accurate information about MS from reputable sources can support informed decision making and contribute to feelings of empowerment. This information provides a language for talking with family, friends, and coworkers about MS. Keep in mind that not everyone learns at the same rate or in the same way. While information can reduce worry for some people, too much information can increase worry for others. Also, some people prefer learning on their own while others prefer learning in a group such as an educational program sponsored by one of the MS organizations or pharmaceutical companies. It's important to respect these differences.

Effective communication skills—Focusing on listening as well as talking, learning to be clear and specific when asking for help, letting people know their help is appreciated, and clarifying what people are saying rather than assuming are all aspects of good communication.

Effective stress management—This process starts with identifying the sources of stress and then prioritizing the stressors so that efforts aimed at stress reduction can be targeted. Keep in mind that MS is often not the primary source of stress for the person with MS or support partners. In many cases, MS doesn't even make the top three sources of stress. It can also be helpful to identify the effects of stress. For example, some people, when stressed, are more likely to be affected physically and experience muscle tension and discomfort in their head, neck, shoulders, and back. Others notice their mood is not as good and they are more irritable, short-tempered, or down in the dumps when stressed. For many people, their behavior is different when they are stressed. They are more likely to lose their temper and engage in unhealthy behaviors such as eating, smoking, drinking, and shopping. Effective stress management includes taking care of basic needs including good sleep, healthy eating, regular exercise, and involvement with people.

Spending time in relaxing activities alone or with supportive people can provide positive distractions from stress. These are all potential tools for that toolbox.

Dealing with emotional distress—This includes acknowledging and talking about feelings, both informally with family and friends and formally with a mental health professional, when symptoms of depression and anxiety are making life with MS even more difficult.

Problem-solving skills—This is a process that involves several steps including defining the problem accurately, generating several options for what might help, and trying one out. After trying an option, it helps to evaluate how well it worked while being willing to try something else if the problem is still just as big.

Flexibility—This refers to being willing to do something in a different way, at a different time of day, with assistance, for shorter periods of time, spread over several days rather than one, and/or with assistive equipment.

Realistic goal setting—Goals that are relatively small, specific, and measureable (a person can tell when the goal has been completed) are more likely to be accomplished. Small, realistic, and achievable goals are less likely to result in people feeling overwhelmed and tend to motivate them to keep trying.

Courage—This means trying something in spite of fear rather than waiting until there is no fear.

Seeking professional help—People who cope more effectively are likely to realize they can't do it alone. They seek services from the members of their health care team, but they serve as the captain on this MS team.

WHAT CAN I DO?

Remember to think:

- Challenge rather than threat

- Difficult but not impossible

- Reduction of difficulties rather than elimination of difficulties

- Adaptation, accommodation, and adjustment rather than acceptance

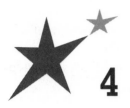

4 Mood and Cognition

Rosalind Kalb and Ann Mullinix

INTRODUCTION

When people hear the words "multiple sclerosis," the picture that generally comes to mind is of someone who has difficulty walking and uses some kind of tool or mobility aid to move around. While it's true that mobility problems are common in MS, people are often surprised to learn that changes in mood and thinking (cognition) are common too. This chapter describes what we know about the psychological changes that can occur, and provides recommendations for how to recognize them, manage them, and explain them to others. Taking charge of mood and cognitive symptoms not only makes life easier and more comfortable, but significantly increases a person's ability to manage the day-to-day challenges of MS and participate effectively in his or her own care.

DEPRESSION AND OTHER MOOD CHANGES

Depression

Depression is common in people with MS—more common than in the general population or in other chronic illnesses. The current thinking is that depression in MS is caused by a combination of factors, including damage in areas of the brain that influence mood, immune system changes, and the changes and losses that often characterize life with

MS—in other words, a triple whammy. What this means is that depression in MS is not about being weak or wimpy, it's about having a mood-related symptom that is as deserving of accurate diagnosis and treatment as any other symptom that can occur. And the risks associated with untreated depression are significant. Depression is known to:

- Reduce a person's quality of life
- Make other symptoms feel worse
- Affect thinking, concentration, and memory
- Decrease participation and productivity
- Interfere with relationships
- Increase a person's risk of suicide

Recognizing Depression

Given the impact depression can have, one would think it would be easy to recognize—but it isn't always. Like everything else with MS, each person's experience is likely to feel a little different and look a little different from everyone else's experience. So let's start by defining what depression is. All of us have down days when we feel sad, discouraged, or blue. In this chapter, however, we are talking about *major depressive disorder* or *clinical depression*.

Symptoms of Clinical Depression

A person with this kind of depression experiences five or more of the following symptoms—almost non-stop—for at least two weeks:

- Ongoing feelings of depression, irritability, or both
- Loss of interest or pleasure in just about everything
- Rapid, significant, and unintentional weight change—either down or up

(continued)

Symptoms of Clinical Depression (*continued*)

■ *Changes in sleep patterns, including difficulty falling or staying asleep, or sleeping much more than usual

■ *Behavior that appears either very agitated to others or very slowed

■ *Ongoing fatigue or loss of energy

■ *Reduced ability to think, concentrate, or make decisions

■ Thoughts of worthlessness or extreme guilt

■ Recurrent thoughts of death or suicide or a suicide attempt

The list sounds pretty straightforward, but there are several reasons why depression often goes unrecognized in MS.

■ Several of the key symptoms of depression (marked above with an *) can also be symptoms of MS, so it may be difficult to tell the difference. People with MS may appear to move or act more slowly, have disturbed sleep, feel very tired, and have problems with thinking or concentration without being at all depressed.

■ In MS, depression often appears as excessive irritability or moodiness, rather than the more typical despair and irrational feelings of guilt—making it difficult for people with MS or their support partners to recognize it.

■ People may be unwilling to acknowledge mood changes because they don't want to be seen as weak or "crazy."

■ A person who has multiple physical limitations as a result of MS may not want to acknowledge that MS can also affect mood.

■ Depression may be difficult to distinguish from the normal grieving process that accompanies the changes and losses caused by MS.

■ Although people are most susceptible to depression at points of major change (at diagnosis, following significant loss of function, or in the midst of a major life change or change in roles), depression can occur at any time—even before the onset of physical symptoms of MS.

For all these reasons, the diagnosis of depression is best made by a health care professional. Any person who experiences a major shift in mood that lasts for at least two weeks without improvement should share this information with his or her physician or nurse so that the problem can be accurately diagnosed and a referral made to the appropriate mental health professional. Even if the person is not experiencing symptoms severe enough to meet the criteria for a diagnosis of major depression, he or she may still be feeling a significant amount of emotional pain and discomfort that would benefit from treatment.

Treating Depression

Depression is one of the most treatable symptoms of MS. Yet we know from extensive research in this area that depression in MS is not being adequately diagnosed or adequately treated. Given how often most people with MS see a physician, it's reasonable to ask why depression is such a neglected symptom.

■ Too often, depression is taken for granted in people with a chronic illness: "I have MS—of course I'm depressed!" or "Who wouldn't be depressed with a disease like that?" or "All my MS patients are depressed—why wouldn't they be?" But clinical depression is never "normal," and it is not an inevitable part of life with MS—prompt diagnosis and treatment can relieve pain and distress and improve quality of life, even in the face of a chronic illness.

■ "Don't ask, don't tell" seems to be a common phenomenon. During the limited time doctors have with patients these days, many simply don't ask about mood symptoms or mood changes. This may be because of time constraints or because they don't feel comfortable or competent in dealing with psychological symptoms. In some parts of the country, physicians may not address emotional issues because they don't have appropriate specialists to whom they can refer their patients. And many patients either don't know that this is an appropriate subject for discussion with the medical team, or are too embarrassed or ashamed to mention it. Unfortunately, too many people worry about being "good patients" ("I don't want to disappoint him ... I don't want her to think less of me ... I don't want to bother her with this"), leaving their concerns about mood at the door.

■ When depression is diagnosed in someone with MS, it is often under-treated. Although neurologists, internists, and family practice physicians may feel comfortable making the diagnosis of depression and starting a patient on treatment, they often don't have the time or expertise to do the follow-up needed to determine if the treatment is working adequately, if the dosage needs to be increased, or if the side effects are well-tolerated. As a result many people stop taking the medication because it hasn't provided sufficient relief or is making them too uncomfortable.

■ In addition, the prescribing physician may never have emphasized the importance of combining medication with psychotherapy and exercise to manage the depression most effectively. Research and clinical experience have clearly shown that all three contribute to the effective management of depression. Medication addresses the changes in the brain that are associated with depression; psychotherapy provides support, problem-solving strategies, and coping skills; and exercise elevates mood—a pretty unbeatable combination.

■ Although self-help groups and social media can provide support and comfort for people who are depressed, they are not sufficient to treat a major depression. Once someone has been adequately diagnosed and treated, they can put these in-person and online support options to better use.

■ Many people with MS take so many medications that they are unwilling to consider taking another—until a trial of medication clearly demonstrates its life-changing benefits.

Tips for Dealing With Depression

Given the challenges to diagnosing and treating depression, it's important for people with MS and their support partners to take charge of this aspect of MS care. Learning about possible mood changes in MS is a critical first step (see Recommended Resources at the end of the chapter).

Managing Mood Issues

People with MS are encouraged to:

■ Pay attention to changes in their mood

■ Bring them to the attention of their physician or nurse

■ Request a referral for an evaluation by a mental health professional with expertise in MS or chronic illness.

■ Be open to a trial of medication if needed, and stick with it long enough for the medication to take effect (up to six weeks or more for an antidepressant, for example).

■ Keep in mind that there are many effective medications available to treat depression and other mood changes. If one doesn't work, or causes uncomfortable side effects (for example, weight gain, stomach upset, sexual dysfunction), there are others to be tried. The treatment of mood changes is as much an art as a science; it may take time and patience to find the most effective treatment or combination of treatments to achieve a sufficient benefit.

■ Remember that the corticosteroids that are commonly prescribed to treat MS relapses can have a significant impact on mood. People may feel highly energized while on steroids—even a bit "wired"—only to experience an emotional slump as they come off them. For some, the mood changes can be extreme and uncomfortable and should be reported promptly to one's health care professional.

Support partners are encouraged to:

■ Pay attention and speak up if they notice changes in their partner.

■ Recognize that depression is not a sign of weakness or "giving in"; encouraging or expecting a loved one to "tough it out," "get a grip," or "be strong," is unrealistic in

(continued)

Managing Mood Issues (*continued*)

the face of significant depression, and may actually get in the way of the necessary diagnosis and treatment.

■ Encourage the person to seek an evaluation. If someone is worried about disappointing or worrying family members, encouragement by their support partners can make it easier to acknowledge the problem and take action.

■ Make every effort not to take their partner's irritability or withdrawal personally. While it can be extremely painful to be on the receiving end of this kind of behavior, it likely has less to do with the relationship than with the depression.

■ Pay attention to their own mood. Mood changes aren't contagious; however for different but equally compelling reasons, support partners are also at risk for depression.

OTHER MOOD CHANGES IN MS

Anxiety

Anxiety, like depression, is extremely common in individuals with MS. This isn't surprising, given the unpredictability of the disease course and the symptoms MS can cause, and the fact that we have no cure for MS at this time, but anxiety is no less deserving of diagnosis and treatment than depression. Severe anxiety that interferes with a person's ability to manage the disease and other important aspects of daily life, to utilize effective problem-solving strategies, or to maintain relationships with family, friends, and colleagues can and should be treated.

Recognizing Anxiety

Since feeling anxious is a normal, expectable response to situations that feel scary, unpredictable, or out of control, it may be difficult to figure out when it's time to seek out help. Some signs that the anxiety is getting in a person's way might include:

■ A preoccupation with scary thoughts that interferes with daily activities or nighttime rest, but doesn't ever seem to lead to productive problem-solving. Some people become so overwhelmed by "what-ifs" (I end up in a wheelchair . . . can't do my job . . . lose my vision . . . end up in a nursing home . . . develop problems with my memory or thinking) that they can't perform on the job or in their household, engage in enjoyable activities with family or friends, or focus their attention on anything else.

■ An increase in physical discomforts—headaches, gastrointestinal problems, heart pounding or palpitations—which are unexplained by other health issues. Since headaches and other uncomfortable sensations can be related to MS, it's important to discuss them and any other significant changes with the health care team in order to determine which might be related to MS, which might signal the presence of other health issues, and which might be the result of anxiety or stress.

Treating Anxiety

Many different interventions can be helpful in relieving anxiety:

■ Self-help groups may offer people the opportunity to share their fears and concerns with others who may experience them. In this kind of supportive environment, individuals can exchange effective problem-solving strategies, suggest community resources, and recognize that they are not alone in their efforts to manage life with MS. For many people, this group experience is enough to take the edge off their anxiety.

■ Individual counseling provides a means for people to face their greatest fears head on and problem-solve around them. In other words, the therapy can help those who are immobilized by their anxiety to feel more in control and more prepared to take positive steps to address the things they fear. If, for example, a woman is frightened about the possibility of being unable to work in the future because of her MS, the therapy might focus on strategies to help her stay productively employed, beginning with steps she can take now to educate herself about her MS, the laws that are designed to protect her rights in the workplace, and the resources she could tap to help her maintain employment in the event she becomes significantly disabled by her MS. Rather than continuing to lose sleep over financial worries, she might follow the therapist's recommendations to consult a financial planner in order to learn strategies for protecting her financial future in the event she becomes unable to work. By becoming educated and taking steps to feel more prepared, she has created enough of a safety net for herself that she's no longer preoccupied by her fears.

■ Sometimes the anxiety is severe enough to prevent a person from being able to make the most of this kind of counseling experience. For anxiety of this severity, medication may be the recommended first step. Once the anxiety is reduced, the person can begin to address the issues in a productive, problem-solving way.

Tips for Dealing With Anxiety

Having a chronic illness does not mean that one has to live with intolerable anxiety. Reporting these uncomfortable feelings to the health care team is the first step to feeling better. People with MS and their support partners are susceptible to significant anxiety so it is important they encourage each other to get the help they need.

Irritability and Temper Outbursts

In addition to the irritability that can occur with depression, there are people with MS who describe moodiness or irritability that feels out of control and out of character. They find themselves snapping at people, losing their temper in inappropriate ways, feeling impatient and out of sorts in a way that is new for them. In situations that are annoying or frustrating, they feel less able to control their responses than they used to.

53

And their family members and colleagues describe them as cranky, prickly, and difficult to be with. It is important for several reasons for the person with MS or family members to report these kinds of changes to the health care team. Since irritability can be a sign of depression, the most important reason is to determine if depression might be the cause. If depression is ruled out, there are other strategies to address this irritability that seems to stem from some combination of neurological changes caused by MS and the daily challenges created by the disease. Medication can be used to help a person feel more in control and more like his or her "old self." In addition, counseling—often including family members—can help everyone understand why the irritability or outbursts are occurring and offer strategies for handling them more comfortably.

Pseudobulbar Affect

Pseudobulbar affect (PBA) refers to uncontrolled episodes of crying and/or laughing that are caused by damage in areas of the brain that control the expression of emotion. The hallmark of this condition, which occurs in MS as well as other neurologic diseases, is that the laughing and crying are unrelated to the person's feelings or are totally out of proportion to the present situation. In other words, a person might begin to cry uncontrollably without having any feelings of sadness or without being in a sad situation. Or a person might begin to laugh uncontrollably even when nothing is funny. These uncontrolled outbursts of emotion are embarrassing to the individual and confusing to others—often leading to problems at home and in the workplace.

Fortunately, PBA is not extremely common in MS. It occurs in about 10 percent of people and can be successfully managed in most. In 2010, a medication called Nuedexta (dextromenthophan + quinidine) was approved to treat PBA in people with MS and other neurologic conditions. The greatest obstacle to treatment of this condition is lack of awareness on the part of people with MS, family members, and health care providers. Prompt reporting of puzzling, uncontrolled episodes of crying or laughing to the health care team is the first step to effective treatment. Education and support for people with PBA and their family members can help promote understanding and successful management of the episodes.

Finding Mental Health Resources

Depression and other mood issues are best treated by a mental health professional with expertise in MS. Unfortunately this kind of specialist may not be as readily available in rural areas as in urban areas. The National MS Society (800-344-4867) can provide referrals to clinicians who are knowledgeable about mood issues in MS. Mental health providers include:

- **Psychiatrists**—Physicians (MD's) who provide diagnosis and treatment. All can prescribe medications and some also provide psychotherapy.

- **Psychiatric nurses**—Nurses with specialized training in diagnosing and treating mood issues. Some psychiatric nurses are licensed to prescribe medication while others are not.

- **Psychologists**—Clinicians with a PhD or MA degree who diagnose mood issues and provide individual, family, and group psychotherapy. Although some psychologists are licensed in their state to prescribe psychiatric medications, most are not. Psychologists may also be engaged in research about mood and other psychosocial issues.

- **Social workers**—Licensed clinicians with a social work degree who focus on providing psychotherapy for individuals and families. Social workers also help to connect people with valuable resources, including essential community programs and services.

- **Counselors**—Clinicians who are licensed to provide counseling services to individuals and families. Counselors may specialize in mental health counseling, marriage and family counseling, vocational counseling, rehabilitation counseling, or other specialties.

Cognitive Changes in MS

The word "cognition" refers to many different kinds of high-level functions related to thinking and memory. Although MS-related cognitive changes were recognized more than 160 years ago, it wasn't until fairly recently that they became the focus of attention by people with MS, health care professionals, and researchers. Today, they are the subject of more intensive research than virtually any other MS symptom. And there are several important reasons for this; changes in a person's ability to think clearly and remember effectively can:

■ Threaten a person's self-esteem and self-confidence

■ Reduce productivity and efficiency

■ Increase the risk of job loss

■ Interfere with communication

■ Alter others' perceptions of, and confidence in, the person's abilities

■ Alter the balance in a relationship based on collaboration, shared responsibilities, and mutual trust

Like other symptoms of MS, cognitive changes are highly variable from one person to another and over time for the same individual. We know that approximately half of people with MS will experience some change in their cognition over the course of the illness. While cognitive dysfunction is somewhat more common in progressive forms of MS, these changes can occur at any point—even as the very first symptom of MS! And although cognitive changes have been found to correlate with total lesion area and tissue loss (atrophy) in the brain, they have a very low correlation with a person's level of physical disability—so that a person with few or no physical symptoms can have extensive cognitive challenges while a person who is severely physically disabled may have no cognitive challenges at all. For example, it is possible that a man who is so severely disabled by his MS that he can move only his head and mouth can be a professor of mathematics at a large university. It is also possible that a young woman with no physical symptoms of MS can experience cognitive symptoms that significantly interfere with her ability to work or live independently. What this means, of course, is that family members, friends, colleagues, and even health care professionals can't tell by looking at a person with MS whether he or she is having cognitive problems. Thus, a significant challenge for people who have experienced cognitive changes is deciding whether, when, and how to explain these invisible changes to others. As with other MS symptoms, the more quickly these changes are reported to the health care team, the more efficiently they can be diagnosed, and the more effectively they can be managed.

Recognizing the Types of Cognitive Changes That Can Occur in MS

- **Memory for recent events**—People with MS-related memory problems may:
  - Have difficulty learning new information and need more time to make the information stick
  - Forget recent conversations, story lines, and characters in a book, TV show, or movie
  - Forget appointments or other plans
  - Lose or misplace things

- **Attention and concentration**—Problems with attention may include:
  - Difficulty staying focused on a task without getting distracted
  - Difficulty multitasking—for example, listening to a family member while cooking
  - Tendency to run out of steam when trying to concentrate on reading material or other intellectual tasks

- **Speed of information processing**—A slowing of thought processes that may be characterized by:
  - Decreased output in spite of time spent and effort exerted (A phenomenon a person might describe as "a brain full of molasses," or "nothing is automatic anymore; I have to think everything through one slow step at a time.")
  - Inability to respond quickly or at all in a rapid-fire conversation or in the face of a lot of simultaneous stimuli (For example, a noisy or complicated environment like a busy restaurant or a lively family dinner, or driving in a high-traffic area with the radio on.)

- Difficulty dealing with tasks having a time element, including projects with deadlines and certain types of games

■ **Executive Functioning**—Problems with executive functions typically include:
   - Inability to plan, prioritize, and organize effectively
   - Difficulty following complex arguments or explanations or missing the point in conversations
   - Trouble following through with multi-step tasks
   - Being too literal or concrete—unable to think abstractly or generalize
   - Difficulty organizing time and meeting deadlines

■ **Visual/spatial organization**—People with visual/spatial problems may:
   - Get lost or disoriented, even in familiar environments
   - Find it difficult to interpret maps or diagrams
   - Have trouble operating devices such as electronic equipment and machinery

■ **Verbal fluency/word finding**—Fluency problems in MS most often include:
   - Word-finding difficulties
   - Getting "lost" or losing one's train of thought while speaking

A person may experience one or more of these difficulties to varying degrees. Once a person has begun to experience cognitive changes, they are unlikely to disappear completely; fortunately, however, the changes generally progress very slowly. Among those with MS who develop cognitive symptoms, most will have relatively mild to moderate problems. A very small percentage of people develop cognitive challenges that are severe enough to cause major disruptions in daily life.

Diagnosing Cognitive Symptoms

Sometimes it is the person with MS who recognizes that she or he doesn't feel as sharp or isn't remembering as well or thinking as clearly as before. Sometimes it's a spouse or partner who picks up on the changes first. And sometimes—unfortunately—it's an employer. In the best of all possible worlds, a person brings any changes to the attention of the health care team sooner rather than later, so that steps can be taken to assess and pinpoint the problems and implement strategies to deal with them. Some common obstacles to diagnosis and treatment include:

■ Many people don't bring the problem to their doctor's attention, either because they are unaware that MS can cause cognitive problems or because they're so frightened about the possibility of cognitive changes that they're reluctant to acknowledge or discuss them.

■ Many doctors incorrectly believe that the Mini Mental State Exam that's included in the neurologic exam (for example, asking the patient to remember three words, count or recite the alphabet backwards, name the President) is sufficient to identify a person with cognitive problems. However, research has shown that the mental status exam will miss at least 50 percent of people with difficulties.

■ Health care professionals may be unaware of the relationship between MS and cognition or may be unsure what to do for someone who is experiencing changes.

■ Some clinicians may be reluctant to ask their patients about cognitive issues because there are limited treatment options available in the community.

■ Anyone above the age of 50 or so is likely to hear from their peers, "Oh don't worry about it—that happens to me all the time!" which may delay their decision to report changes to the health care professional.

In light of these potential obstacles, people with MS will need to advocate on their own behalf in order to get these symptoms adequately assessed and treated. The assessment of cognitive problems is usually done by a neuropsychologist (a psychologist with special training in the assessment and treatment of cognitive functioning), an occupational therapist, or a speech/language pathologist. While these clinicians utilize different tests for evaluating cognition, they share an interest in identifying areas of difficulty and areas of strength, and assessing the impact of cognitive challenges on everyday life.

The first step in any evaluation should be to evaluate the person for depression. Since depression is known to affect cognitive function, adequately treating a person's depression may significantly improve cognitive performance.

Cognitive evaluations range from brief screening batteries that highlight possible problems, to lengthy (6–8 hours) test batteries that carefully evaluate each cognitive function in order to identify areas of change or loss and areas of strength. Identifying areas of strength is extremely important because the primary goal of treatment is to help people learn how to utilize their cognitive strengths to compensate for any cognitive changes that might have occurred. For example, a person who more easily remembers things he or she has seen than things that have been heard will learn to make notes, post reminders, and take advantage of all available visual cues.

A cognitive assessment is particularly important for anyone who:

■ Has experienced changes that are interfering with everyday activities and/or important relationships

■ Is concerned about job performance or has received a negative job evaluation

■ Is considering applying for Society Security Disability Insurance (SSDI). Cognition is one of the four criteria, along with vision, walk- ing ability, and fatigue, which are considered by the Social Security Administration for people with MS.

■ Is worried about the possibility of cognitive changes in the future and would like to have a baseline assessment

Treating Cognitive Changes

At the present time, we have no medications that have been shown in controlled clinical trials to treat or cure cognitive dysfunction in people with MS. As already mentioned, however, an antidepressant may be helpful for someone whose cognitive changes are primarily due to depression. Similarly, a medication used to treat fatigue might help someone whose cognition is primarily affected by MS-related fatigue.

The MS disease-modifying therapies may be the most effective way to delay or slow the progression of cognitive changes. Since cognitive changes are related to the amount of damage in the brain, and the disease-modifying therapies help to reduce the number of MS relapses and lesions on magnetic resonance imaging (MRI), it stands to reason that taking one of these medications might reduce a person's risk of worsening cognitive symptoms. While there is as of yet insufficient evidence to prove that connection, it certainly could be considered another good reason to start on treatment early in the disease.

Cognitive rehabilitation is the most promising strategy at this time to manage MS-related cognitive changes. In sessions with a neuropsychologist, occupational therapist, or speech/language pathologist, a person can learn compensatory strategies that are specifically tailored to his or her cognitive difficulties. A prime example of a compensatory strategy is learning how to substitute organization for memory. For example, it's possible to organize a person's workspace and home environment in such a way that things are less likely to get lost; templates can be created to guide the person through the steps involved in carrying out important activities (balancing a checkbook, preparing a meal, going to the grocery store), tools/maps can be devised to help the person navigate without getting lost. The end result is that the individual learns to use a variety of tools in place of the cognitive functions that are no longer working as reliably as they once did. One might compare these strategies to the mobility aids that allow a person to stay active, productive, and engaged even though her or his walking is impaired. Because cognitive changes in MS tend to progress slowly, the best strategy is learning how to compensate early on, when the learning is easier and faster. Once good compensatory strategies are in place, it's possible to tweak them as the person's needs change.

WHAT CAN I DO?

The essential first step is to decide that it's OK to do things a little differently than in the past.

Strategies for Getting Organized

■ Get rid of scraps of paper and scattered Post-It® notes; keep all your important information in a centralized place

(continued)

Strategies for Getting Organized (*continued*)

- A daily planner, paper or electronic, is a great tool for time management, contact numbers, important medical information, and daily reminder notes

- Set up and maintain a filing system that makes sense to you

- Insist on a family calendar to keep track of everyone's activities and appointments

- Have a specific place for easily-lost items like keys, glasses, TV remotes

- Put clear labels on filing cabinets, storage boxes

- Process incoming mail daily and keep all bills in the same place

- Create a system for phone messages

- Create a consistent routine; perform the same tasks on the same days of the week

- Use a timer to keep track of when to stop/start activities

- Clean out clutter and simplify your living space; physical clutter is mind clutter

Strategies to Deal With Memory Problems

- Substitute organization for memory

- Our minds find it easiest to remember groupings of one to three items (think of how phone numbers are grouped)

- Use paper or electronic organizers, calendars, computers, GPS systems

- Set alarms on phones or computers to remind yourself of appointments, when to start dinner, or when to rest

(continued)

Strategies to Deal With Memory Problems (*continued*)

- Make sure to return items to their designated spot
- Use checklists (grocery lists, to-do lists, birthday lists)
- Try not to multitask; focus on one thing at a time in order to retain information more easily
- Reinforce memory by talking out loud; repeat and associate bits of information
- When away from home or work, leave voice messages for yourself, or use a micro-recorder that is small enough to fit into a purse or backpack; if it is inconvenient to write or use a recorder for reminders, moving one's watch to the opposite wrist can serve as a reminder
- Reduce environmental distractions as much as possible

Strategies to Enhance Attention and Concentration

- Create quiet, distraction-free places for important conversations and tasks
- Identify sources and patterns of distraction at home and work
- Work on the most difficult tasks when feeling most rested and refreshed
- Pace your work with regular rest breaks
- Take regular visual rest breaks when using the computer; look away after every 15 minutes of use
- Use high contrast, large font, anti-glare computer screens, and good lighting to lessen impact of visual changes and mental fatigue

Utilizing the Health Care Team

Physical therapist—Research has shown that exercise can improve mood and may improve cognitive function as well. Check with your physician and physical therapist about the kinds of exercise that would be best for you.

Neurologist or nurse—During the busy office visit, it is difficult to cover all the important issues you may be dealing with. Be sure to mention any concerns you have about mood changes or cognitive problems so that your health care team can work with you to get them properly diagnosed and treated.

Occupational therapist—It is easy to become frustrated, anxious, angry, and be hard on oneself with cognitive challenges. Relax. Step away from a task that is going nowhere and give yourself some "mental space." Take a deep breath. Meditation is a dynamic approach for calming, increasing awareness, and improving attention and concentration. A good start for meditation is working on awareness of the breath and deep breathing from the belly. For example, breathe in for a count of five, pause, then release for another count of five. Repeat this five times. This simple technique can be done anywhere at almost any time. The goal of belly breathing is to promote inner calmness, clarity, and mental energy.

WHAT CAN I DO?

- Keep a tool kit ready for immediate use. Having prepared statements such as, "I will get back to you on that," or having a pen and small notebook readily available can make situations more comfortable and can reduce the stress that certainly doesn't help memory.

- Allow yourself to ask for clarification, reminders, directions, and assistance. Learn your limits and when to say "no."

- Overall, it is best to start small, try one technique that realistically can fit into your daily life and try it for 2 to 4 weeks. Any cognitive strategy must have intrinsic value to motivate us to be effective. Remember, you can still do it; you may just need to be more mindful in going through the process of obtaining, organizing, and retrieving information.

RECOMMENDED RESOURCES

Books

Farrell, P. (2011). *It's Not All in Your Head: Depression, Anxiety, and Mood Swings and MS*. New York: Demos Medical Publishing.

Gingold, J. (2011). *Facing the Cognitive Challenges of Multiple Sclerosis*. 2nd ed. New York: Demos Medical Publishing.

Gingold, J. (2009). *Mental Sharpening Stones: Manage the Cognitive Challenges of Multiple Sclerosis*. New York: Demos Medical Publishing.

Kabat-Zinn, J. (1990). *Full Catastrophe Living: Using the Wisdom of Your Body and Mind to Face Stress, Pain, and Illness*. New York: Delacorte Press.

LaRocca, N., and R. Kalb. (2006). *Multiple Sclerosis: Understanding the Cognitive Challenges*. New York: Demos Medical Publishing.

Schwarz, S. P. (2006). *Multiple Sclerosis: 300 Tips for Making Life Easier*. 2nd ed. New York: Demos Medical Publishing.

Shadday, A. (2007). *MS and Your Feelings: Handling the Ups and Downs of Multiple Sclerosis*. Alameda, CA: Hunter House.

Websites

Portable Health Profile: Courage Center of Minneapolis, MN—a site to help you keep track of your health records. http://www.couragecenter.org/images/documents/Portable%20Health%20Profile.pdf

AbleData.com—A website listing more than 20,000 assistive technology products, With descriptions, prices, ordering information, and installation instructions.

From the National MS Society

Mood

Depression and Multiple Sclerosis—an 11-page brochure on recognizing and management depression. http://www.nationalmssociety.org/download.aspx?id=53

Multiple Sclerosis and Your Emotions—a 23-page booklet that discusses mood changes and the role of stress. http://www.nationalmssociety.org/download.aspx?id=151

MS Learn Online programs: health grieving, depression, anxiety, pseudobulbar affect. http://www.nationalmssociety.org/multimedia-library/ms-learn-online/ms-learn-online-healthy-living/index.aspx#Feature Presentations

Cognition

Solving Cognitive Problems—a 24-page booklet about strategies to manage cognitive changes. http://www.nationalmssociety.org/download. aspx?id=61

Hold that Thought: Cognition and MS—a 50-page book about the diagnosis and management of cognitive changes in ms. http://www. nationalmssociety.org/download.aspx?id=1392

CogniFitness: Keeping the Mind Moving—an 8-week course offered through chapters of the National MS Society for restorative and compensatory skill training for cognitive challenges.

Accessible Technology—information about assistive technology tools to help with cognitive challenges. www.nationalmssociety.org/Assistive Technology

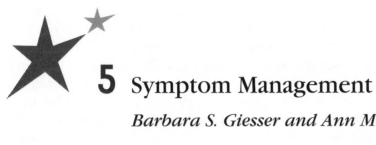

5 Symptom Management

Barbara S. Giesser and Ann Mullinix

A person who was diagnosed with MS a generation ago was likely to encounter the "diagnose and adios" approach. They might have been offered steroids if they were having an acute attack, and generally were told to go home and "take it easy" and call their doctor if they needed an assistive device. There was no therapy that could be used to reduce relapses or slow progression, and few symptomatic treatments. People were commonly told to avoid exercise, and not to have children, and sometimes ended up becoming more disabled by (well meaning but inaccurate) neurologic advice, than by their neurologic condition.

Fortunately, the past two decades have seen remarkable advances in knowledge about and treatments for MS. The current state of the art management for persons with MS combines disease modifying treatments (DMTs) with a comprehensive approach to addressing symptoms. There are also important new findings about the roles of exercise and lifestyle changes that can help persons with MS live optimally with their disease.

DMTs are medications that work by changing the underlying immune dysfunction that is widely thought to be responsible for producing the nerve damage that occurs in MS. The first DMT approved to treat MS was released in 1993. There are eight FDA approved DMTs and several in large scale clinical trials. These medications have definitively demonstrated that they reduce the frequency and severity of relapses, reduce the occurrence of new and inflamed areas of nerve damage as seen on MRI scans ("lesions"), and in some cases slow disease progression. These medications have allowed people with MS to go for long periods of time disease free, and have made a profound difference in the way persons with MS and their neurologists can approach the disease. The DMTs make it possible to be proactive, and minimize nerve damage and attacks, instead of merely reacting to them when they occur. By the time someone is diagnosed with MS, the disease process has already been present for some time, and has most likely produced nerve damage that cannot even be seen yet on MRI. Also, once nerve damage has occurred it is usually permanent. Most neurologists believe that treatment with DMTs should be started early, as soon as a definite diagnosis of MS is confirmed.

Choosing a DMT is a very individual decision that ideally is arrived at with input from both the person with MS and their physician. There is no one "best" agent and no "one size fits all" approach. Things to consider when choosing a DMT include the efficacy and tolerability of the drug, routes of administration and short term and long term potential side effects.

DMTs significantly reduce exacerbations but do not stop them entirely. An MS attack or exacerbation is conventionally defined as the appearance of new neurologic symptoms, or the return or worsening of a pre-existing symptom, that lasts at least 24 to 48 hours. If an exacerbation does not resolve promptly on its own, or more importantly, interferes with the person's ability to carry out their usual routine, then it is most commonly treated with a brief course of oral or intravenous corticosteroids. Rehabilitative treatments may be needed as well. If the attack is thought to have a cause, usually an infection or becoming overheated, then it is called a "pseudo exacerbation" and usually resolves when the underlying infection is treated or a cooling strategy is applied.

Although those living with MS who are treated with DMTs have fewer relapses, DMTs do **not** treat symptoms. Even in periods of "remission"—the time when new symptoms are less pronounced—the person may still have substantial inconvenience or difficulty in functioning from the many common symptoms associated with MS. Management with DMTs goes hand in hand with symptom management. DMTs help people with MS have periods of attack-free stability. Managing symptoms ensures that people feel and function at their best.

Treatment with DMTs, and the role of the neurologist in general, is just one piece of the puzzle in MS management. Almost all the symptoms that MS can cause respond best to a combination of medication, rehabilitative strategies, and lifestyle modifications. Fortunately, there are health care professionals with expertise in MS in all the disciplines that a person with MS might need to access. These include physical medicine and rehabilitation physicians, nurses, physician assistants, physical therapists (PTs), occupational therapists (OTs), speech/language pathologists, mental health professionals, dieticians, social workers and exercise physiologists. Also, physicians from other medical specialties, such as urology, gynecology, or psychiatry may be called upon to add their expertise to management as well.

Another very important resource for the person with MS to call upon in managing their MS is their support partner. Many symptoms of MS are "invisible" such as fatigue, pain, or spasticity and may not be readily apparent, but can cause significant problems. A support partner, who is familiar with these and can recognize them, can help the person with MS deal with them most effectively. Support partners also can help the person with MS adhere to medication regimens, provide an additional set of ears when going to the provider, and may often relay important information to any of the health care professionals that the person with MS may not recognize in themselves.

MULTIPLE APPROACHES CAN BE USED TO MANAGE MANY SYMPTOMS

The most common symptom seen in people with MS is fatigue. Some studies have reported that 90 percent of persons with MS experience fatigue at some time. MS fatigue differs from "normal" fatigue in that it may come on suddenly, tends to be worse with heat, is not necessarily a result of exertion or poor sleep, and most importantly, interferes with the person's ability to carry out their normal functions. MS fatigue can have many contributing factors and its treatment is multifactorial. We will use fatigue to illustrate an MS symptom that is best treated by a comprehensive approach that combines medical/neurologic, rehabilitative, and lifestyle interventions. When reading about other symptoms, you can refer back to this comprehensive way of addressing treatment with a team approach.

WHAT CAN I DO?

It is a good idea to review all of your medications with your provider to see if there are any that may particularly be a source of fatigue or sedation. Often a substitute may be found or alternate ways of taking them may alleviate this problem.

WHAT CAUSES FATIGUE IN PERSONS WITH MS?

In order to answer this question, it is helpful to divide MS related fatigue into "primary" and "secondary." Primary MS fatigue is not well understood, but is thought to be caused directly by damage to nerves in the brain and spinal cord. Primary MS fatigue is often made worse by other MS symptoms, including pain, weakness, spasticity, and depression, and so treating these other symptoms may need to be concurrently addressed.

Secondary fatigue is related to other factors or conditions that can cause fatigue independently from MS. These include medical, pharmacologic, physiologic, and nutritional problems (Figure 1).

Common medical problems that might cause or worsen fatigue include underactive thyroid or other endocrine problems, anemia, and heart or lung disease. Most of these can be diagnosed with simple lab tests and be appropriately treated. This evaluation is usually done by a primary health care provider in family practice or internal medicine.

Many medications that are used to manage MS can have fatigue or sedation as a side effect. Among DMTs, the beta-interferons often cause fatigue or malaise. Some chemotherapy agents that are sometimes used to treat progressive MS cause fatigue as well.

Among symptom management drugs, the antispasticity medications, including baclofen, tizanidine, and benzodiazepines may commonly be sedating, particularly at higher doses.

Medications used for pain, which include opiates, antiseizure drugs, which include gabapentin or carbamazepine, or antidepressant medications such as amitriptyline, may all be sedating. Often, these agents are taken at night to minimize their sedating effects. Some medications used for other medical conditions, such as certain blood pressure medications, can also produce fatigue or sedation.

Depression can be a significant source of or contributor to fatigue. It is best managed with a combination of medication when appropriate, therapy or behavioral strategies, and exercise. Poor nutrition often contributes to fatigue directly or may contribute indirectly by promoting obesity, which in itself can impact fatigue. Becoming active can certainly cause fatigue or make primary MS fatigue worse. Try to achieve a balance when treating fatigue.

Sleep problems are more common in people with MS than the general population, and clearly can impact fatigue. Common primary sleep disorders include insomnia, restless legs, and sleep apnea and may be treated after a careful sleep history is taken. Secondary causes of poor sleep due to other MS symptoms, such as spasticity, pain, bladder problems, and depression should also be looked for and treated.

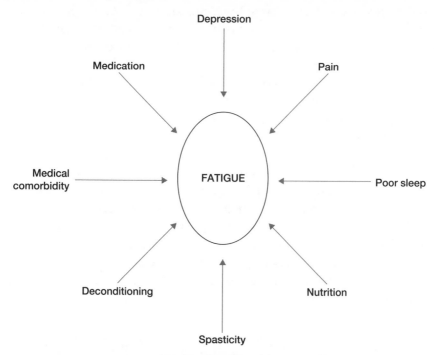

Figure 1 Factors that contribute to fatigue

HOW IS PRIMARY MS FATIGUE TREATED?

Once primary MS fatigue is identified as a problem, a combined team approach is used to treat it.

Medications—There are no medications that have a specific FDA indication to treat MS related fatigue, but several agents are commonly used "off label" for this purpose. Amantadine is a drug that was originally used to prevent viral infections and then was found to help some symptoms of Parkinson's disease. It is most effective for fatigue when it is taken a few hours before the worst fatigue is anticipated. Side effects may include insomnia, dry mouth, or blurry vision. Other agents for fatigue are Provigil® (modafinil) or Nuvigil® (armodafinil). These medications are usually very effective in treating primary MS fatigue but are not always covered by insurance. Side effects may include headache or insomnia. Sometimes central nervous system stimulants may also be tried.

Behavior and lifestyle changes—All people are unique in how fatigue affects their daily lives. Understanding the source of fatigue as mentioned above can guide them in knowing what strategies to use. Learned strategies help stretch energy across an entire day. This lessens the impact of fatigue and increases participation in chosen activities.

These strategies require behavior and lifestyle changes. These changes then become a life practice, promoting wellness and giving hope. As Peggy Crawford stated, learning to deal with challenges creates opportunities to make changes and try new things. This active decision making process encourages participation in activities that are meaningful, making the most of the present day's energy. These powerful strategies are categorized into three groups: mind, body, and environment.

Mind—The mind sets priorities and makes choices. Think of "banking" or saving energy and "budgeting" or spending energy within limits to prevent total depletion. The goal is to always keep a little energy in the bank. Protect this energy by prioritizing activities and balancing activities with rest. Prioritization will allow spending energy on what is important.

Balancing Energy

- Use a daily planner to write each and every activity that needs to be performed during the day.

(continued)

Balancing Energy (*continued*)

- Space activities throughout the day, performing activities that require greater amounts of energy during the time of day you have more energy.

- Learn pacing. Limit time spent on an activity.

- Be flexible.

- Be open to delegating and accepting help.

- Schedule rest.

Rest is the most effective strategy in fighting fatigue:

- Rest before becoming tired.

- Rest does not necessarily mean sleep; it means relaxation. This relaxation may come while reading a book, meditating, or listening to music.

- Napping helps some but it is important that sleep is limited to 20 to 30 minutes, not interfering with sleeping patterns at night.

- Take short, more frequent rest breaks—15 to 20 minutes will help extend energy throughout the day. Pushing through activities to get things done can deplete energy by mid-day.

Body—It is important to be good managers of our health. People with MS are just as prone as the rest of the population to getting other health conditions. Good health is possible even if you have multiple sclerosis.

Increasing Health and Decreasing Fatigue

- Exercise on a regular basis.
- Make dietary changes.

(*continued*)

Increasing Health and Decreasing Fatigue (*continued*)

- Fatigue and stress are interconnected. Implement stress reduction techniques.
- Use larger and stronger muscle groups, such as a shoulder bag instead of a hand purse.
- Avoid straining the body by simplifying its movement.
- Use electrical appliances whenever possible, like a can opener, mixer, or electric toothbrush.
- Use a cart on wheels to transport items such as laundry or groceries.
- Sit to perform such tasks as preparing meals in the kitchen or shaving in the bathroom.
- Move frequently used items in cupboards or closets to within easy reach.
- Keep heavy items, such as a cast iron skillet, on the stovetop.
- Slide heavy objects instead of lifting.
- Remember: push before pull, and pull before lift.
- Use good body mechanics. How one stands and moves saves energy. First, analyze posture. If one stands with the body and head slumped forward and the chin down, shallow breathing occurs. This is not a good use of energy. Posture can be improved by holding the head and neck in alignment with the spine, with the head in a "chin up" position. Relax both shoulders and elongate the spine to place less stress on the body and to promote deeper, energy producing breath.

Environment—Often, we get used to how we perform daily activities and how our home and work environments are organized. Making a few, simple changes to our environments often promotes more efficiency.

Environmental Changes

- Cut down on clutter and simplify the home or work environment.

- Consider temperatures. If on the warm side, use a fan or air conditioner, and if on the cool side, dress in layers to be able to adjust as needed.

- Consider lighting. Frequently used areas should be well lit, yet avoid fluorescent lighting, as some sources claim it can strain eyes and cause mild headaches.

- Be aware of distractions in the environment. Close the door to silence other conversations, and turn off the TV and radio to focus concentration.

- Another modality that is often very effective in relieving fatigue is **cooling.** This can be done simply by applying cold cloths or chewing ice chips, or with more elaborate mechanisms such as cooling garments or hand held cooling devices.

Today there are many different kinds of tools and technology to save energy. As mentioned earlier, using objects with wheels and electrical gadgets gets the job done while saving energy. Adaptive equipment, found at medical supply stores or rehabilitation hospitals, compensate for a change in function yet promote independence. For instance, the loss of hand coordination or strength can challenge many daily living skills. A button hook can more efficiently fasten buttons. When balance is challenged, a reacher can grab items that are out of reach or assist with lower-body dressing. A shower chair allows a person to bathe while seated. A grab bar provides more stability for getting in and out of a shower. A wealth of assistive technology can be used to adapt computers. There seems to be a "gadget" that simplifies a task, saves energy, and promotes independence for almost any daily activity!

Energy management strategies may change the process of how or when activities are performed. However, the end goal is always doing more of what is important. Research shows that incorporating assistive techniques improves daily functioning, quality of life, and confidence.

Rehabilitation professionals such as occupational and physical therapists are specialists who instruct and tailor these strategies to individual needs. Give a few of these strategies a try, and if more assistance is needed, talk to a provider about a referral to a rehabilitation specialist.

Exercise has been demonstrated in many studies to significantly improve fatigue in persons with MS. Definitive guidelines for what types of exercises are best for persons with MS have not been determined, and so exercise regimens need to be developed individually for each person with MS, after consultation with their physician and, ideally, in conjunction with a physical therapist or exercise specialist.

The secondary factors that impact fatigue can also be treated with a combination of pharmacologic and non-pharmacologic strategies. Spasticity, or muscle tightness, responds to medications, stretching, and exercise. Simple nutrition practices such as eating small frequent meals with proteins and complex carbohydrates will help prevent blood sugar crashes and sudden lack of energy. Identifying barriers to sleep, and treating any primary sleep disorders that may exist, such as sleep apnea, will also improve fatigue.

OTHER SYMPTOMS

Common symptoms of MS such as pain, spasticity, and depression occur in most persons with MS at one time or another. Other common symptoms of MS are numbness or tingling, weakness, incoordination, tremor, and visual problems. Disturbances of bladder, bowel, and sexual function may occur in up to 80 percent of persons with MS and are very treatable.

When reading through these symptoms, consider the team approach to management.

Symptom Management: Sensory

The most common sensory symptoms are numbness and tingling or "pins and needles" feelings. Other sensations may be stabbing, lightning or electrical feelings, crawling or itching, or a feeling as though there is a tight band or belt around the torso ("MS hug"). Medications used for these generally include antiseizure medications and some antidepressants. Often, applying local cooling to a painful area is effective.

Symptom Management: Weakness

Muscle weakness can be directly and indirectly attributed to the disease process. MS lesions in the brain or spinal cord directly impair muscle function, and weakness occurs indirectly because a person becomes less active. Pain, spasticity, contractures, a change in sensation, or overusing muscles that are stronger to compensate for weaker muscles, all contribute to secondary or indirect muscle weakness. Acute attacks of weakness with an exacerbation are usually treated with a brief course of corticosteroids.

Rehabilitation professionals such as PT's and OT's work with people to improve strength and compensate for weakness, which helps balance, posture, endurance, and functional independence.

Weakness is managed by incorporating strengthening exercises designed uniquely for each individual, as well as instruction in compensatory techniques. Examples of compensatory techniques are assistive devices for walking, or bracing and adaptive equipment that make daily activities easier. Assistive devices for walking, braces, or other adaptive equipment do not promote disuse or weakness. These devices prevent over-compensating and overuse, while promoting independence, safety, energy management, and reduction of pain.

Symptom Management: Tremors/Ataxia

Tremors may be the most frustrating symptom to overcome and treat. Tremors can interfere with movement, activities of daily living, communication, and eating, and cause increased fatigue. By working with a PT, OT or speech/language pathologist, improvement in function can occur. There are few effective pharmacologic treatments for tremors but some provide benefit so it is worth discussing with your provider.

To reduce tremors, therapists use the concept of weight bearing into the affected body part. For example, eating can be daunting when an arm is in constant motion. Forget what mothers may have taught about not putting elbows on the table. Placing an elbow on the table or placing elbows next to the body will stabilize the arm, lessen movement, and increase control.

 Other Ways to Reduce Tremors

■ Weighted gloves, weighted utensils, or placing light 1 to 2 pound weights around the wrists. It helps to have the arm performing the work in a weight bearing position—on an arm rest, a table, or next to the side—in order for the weights to be effective.

■ Using two hands instead of one can increase strength and control.

■ Sitting with good back support will assist in stabilizing your body.

■ Wearing tighter clothing increases sensory feedback to the brain.

■ Adaptive equipment can be very helpful. Some examples are:
  • Enlarged handles for better hand control.
  • Angled spoons minimize the distance from the plate to your mouth.
  • Right-angle knives cut with less effort.
  • Two handled cups.
  • Dycem, a nonslip material used to secure objects.

Stress and anxiety can negatively impact tremors. If tension is high, taking a few moments to relax and take some deep breaths before resuming the activity will help. Tremors can interfere with eating and drinking adequate amounts. People with MS and family members need to be mindful of that.

Symptom Management: Vision

Vision disturbances in people with MS are common. An acute loss of vision and pain in one eye is called optic neuritis and is the first symptom of MS in about 15 percent of people with MS. This is usually treated with a brief course of corticosteroids. Other symptoms may include blurred or double vision, or bouncing vision. These symptoms may improve over time with or without treatment, but vision changes may be permanent. Many visual symptoms may worsen, though, when a person is overheated or tired, and resolve with rest or cooling.

Compensatory Interventions for Visual Problems

- Increasing contrast:
  - Place duct tape on the edge of each stair (just be sure that the tape color is darker or lighter than the object it is placed on).
  - Highlight lines in books can improve not only seeing words, but also helps with concentration and reducing eye fatigue.
- Decreasing glare:
  - To reduce glare in the environment, wear UV sunglasses or use non-glare screens on computers.
- Improving lighting:
  - When vision is blurry, good lighting throughout the home or work environment improves clarity and contrast.
- Other vision tips:
  - De-clutter environments, place items in the same location at all times.
  - Take visual rest breaks.
  - Enlarged print, magnification, and assistive technology, such as voice activation or screen readers on computers or watches, assist the eyes from overworking.
  - Stores that specialize in low-vision products offer a variety of items that can make the activities in daily life easier.

Some people experience double vision, or diplopia. Patching an eye or using prism glasses made by a neuro-ophthalmologist eliminates seeing double.

Symptom Management: Bowel, Bladder and Sexual Problems

Common symptoms of bladder dysfunction are urinary urgency frequency, hesitancy, getting up to go at night, and frequent bladder infections. Bowel symptoms might include either constipation or loss of bowel control. These problems are easily treated with a combination of medication and other strategies. Exercise helps both bladder and bowel function. Diet and appropriate fluid intake are also important in managing these problems. Discussion with the health care provider is the best starting place for successful management.

Sexual dysfunction in MS is common in both sexes, and can produce erectile dysfunction or vaginal dryness, as well as loss of orgasm, loss of sensation, or painful sensation. Decreased libido is also common. Problems with sexual function may not only be due to MS itself, but can be due to the symptoms of MS such as spasticity, weakness, and pain, and factors such as fatigue, depression, or medication effects. These may be managed by a combination of medication and non-pharmacologic methods. In addition, the social and psychological factors that accompany living with MS may contribute to sexual dysfunction and loss of intimacy.

WHAT CAN I DO?

Very often there is a "don't ask don't tell" attitude about bowel, bladder, and sexual problems. Providers are hesitant to ask, and patients are embarrassed to tell! It is important to tell the provider if there are problems in these areas as they are very successfully treated.

CONCLUSION

The optimal management of MS combines both DMTs and symptom treatment. A comprehensive team approach, incorporating input and strategies from multiple health care disciplines, is the most effective way to alleviate symptoms and empower the person with MS to feel and function at his or her best.

RECOMMENDED READING

Lowenstein, N. (2009). *Fighting Fatigue in Multiple Sclerosis: Practical Ways to Create New Habits and Increase Your Energy.* New York: Demos Medical Publishing.

Mathiowetz, V., K. Matuska, M. Finlayson, P. Luo, and H. Chen. (2007). "One-year Follow-up to a Randomized Controlled Trial of an Energy Conservation Course for Persons with Multiple Sclerosis." *International Journal of Rehabilitation Research 30*: 305–13.

Schwarz, S. P. (2006). *Multiple Sclerosis: 300 Tips for Making Life Easier* (2nd Ed.). New York: Demos Medical Publishing.

Stout, K. (2010). *Fatigue Management in Chronic Illness: Implications for Use in a One-to-One Occupational Therapy Session.* Chicago, IL: Department of Occupational Therapy, University of Illinois.

Stout, K., and M. Finlayson. (2011). "Fatigue Management in Chronic Illness." *OT Practice* 16: 16–19.

RECOMMENDED WEBSITES

The National Multiple Sclerosis Society. http://www.nationalmssociety.org

AbleData, Information on Assistive Technology and Assistive Devices for Daily Living. http://www.abledata.com

Apple Computer Disability Resources. http://apple.com/accessibility/resources/

Microsoft Accessibility Technology for Everyone. http://www.microsoft.com/enable

6 Physical Activity and Exercise Programs

Andrea White, Sue Kushner, and Ann Mullinix

For people with MS, exercise presents opportunities to enhance fitness, health, and well-being. An exercise program may also provide an avenue for social interaction and support. However, there are some challenges associated with exercise for individuals with MS. At this point it is important to distinguish the role of physical activity in MS. The goals of this chapter are focused primarily on how exercise can improve physical fitness and health and how specific types of exercises can be used to maintain specific functions that may be altered by MS. This chapter will incorporate valuable information from an exercise physiologist, a physical therapist (PT) and an occupational therapist (OT). Viewing the topic of exercise from a "team" perspective broadens the aspects of *what* can be done and *how* to best do it.

The U.S. Surgeon General's Report on Physical Activity and Health Findings

- Significant health benefits can be obtained by including a moderate amount of physical activity (30 minutes per day) on most, if not all, days of the week.

(continued)

The U.S. Surgeon General's Report on Physical Activity and Health Findings (*continued*)

■ Physical activity reduces the risk of many chronic conditions including coronary heart disease, hypertension, colon cancer, and diabetes mellitus.

Despite these recommendations, more than 60 percent of American adults are not doing enough physical activity, and 25 percent of all adults are not active at all. Individuals with MS experience many of the health concerns that are associated with being physically inactive and would thus similarly benefit from a well-rounded exercise program. This raises an important question for people who have MS: "If average Americans cannot manage to be physically active, how can we?" Indeed, with mobility constraints, fatigue, and other potential limitations, maintaining an exercise program may seem daunting.

BENEFITS OF EXERCISE IN MS

As recently as the 1990s, individuals with MS were advised not to exercise. It was thought that stress and exposure to higher body temperatures could be harmful. Even so, many people with MS, such as Jimmie Heuga, engaged in regular exercise and found that they felt better. Based on these anecdotal reports, researchers from the Heuga Center for MS (now Can Do Multiple Sclerosis) performed the first controlled study to determine the effects of regular aerobic exercise in people with MS. In this study, 54 patients with MS were randomly assigned to an exercise group or to a non-exercise group. The exercise group experienced significant improvements in aerobic fitness, strength, and mobility. These benefits were not associated with any negative changes in neurological status, and patients even reported that fatigue levels were improved.

Today, there are many published studies related to the beneficial effects of various types of exercise in MS patients. In addition to increasing physical fitness, many other benefits have been identified, including improvements in quality of life. The proactive nature of physical activity, whether it is exercise performed on one's own or in a rehabilitation setting, positively influences quality of life. Studies have shown that general perceptions of health, vitality, and physical and social functioning improved in MS patients who were involved in physical activities such as exercise or other active pursuits such as gardening. Even people with MS who had moderate to severe disability reported positive changes in overall health perception as a result of appropriate exercise. Positive health perceptions were maintained regardless of disease progression. The bottom line is: *Doing something physical is much better than doing nothing.*

FUNCTIONAL RESERVE

In addition to conveying general health benefits, being more fit may increase an individual's ability to withstand the effect of MS relapses. This is the concept of "functional reserve." To illustrate this idea, think of physical function in terms of an amount that you could pour into a water glass that holds 100 units. We can put any type of physical function in this water glass such as walking or swimming. For example, aerobic capacity is a physical function that is related to your ability to do activities that use large muscle groups and increase your heart rate and breathing. Another physical function is your muscular strength and endurance, which relates to how much force you can exert to lift or push things and whether you can keep lifting or pushing for an extended period of time. Now, imagine that in order to perform your necessary daily living tasks and recreational activities, you need your glass to be at least half full (50 units). If a person is healthy and fairly active, his glass may contain 80 units. This means that his "functional reserve" is 30 units (80 minus 50). In other words, this person has 30 units *more* physical function that is necessary just to get by. On the other hand, a person who has been relatively inactive for a long time may have a "glass of function" that contains only 60 units, and as a consequence, their functional reserve is only 10 units.

Now, MS enters the picture. It is possible that a relapse may decrease physical function by 20 units. This may be a short-term decrease, or it may be permanent, depending on how much recovery occurs. According to the examples above, the person with a glass of 80 units will drop to 60 units. Fortunately, this is still well above the functional minimum of 50 units. In contrast, if the inactive person has the same relapse, their volume will decrease from 60 units to 40 units. Having a level below the 50 unit threshold may mean that this person can no longer perform some necessary activities on their own. This could mean that this person can no longer carry in their groceries, or it may mean that the ability to go for a morning walk becomes too difficult. It is possible to be proactive in terms of building reserve by doing some type of physical activity, especially during times that you feel good. The type and amount of activity that is recommended will depend on the physical capabilities and limitations for each individual.

CHALLENGES AND OPPORTUNITIES

Many MS symptoms require that exercise be modified in some way. Loss of sensation, poor position sense, and visual difficulties are common in MS and negatively affect balance and coordination. In addition, fatigue, poor motor control, and mobility constraints can make some forms of exercise difficult and even dangerous.

Many of the challenges individuals with MS face can be overcome by creating a realistic and adaptable exercise plan. Guidance in this process can be obtained in a number of ways. Some communities have ongoing exercise and/or rehabilitation programs sponsored by local MS organizations. Increasingly, fitness leaders at health clubs have experience prescribing exercise to populations with specific needs. It may require a bit of research to locate a program or facility that works, but it is well worth the effort.

Designing an Exercise Program to Improve Health Related Fitness

What Type of Exercise?

■   Aerobic exercise is a major focus because this type of activity conveys many health benefits. Aerobic activities are those that increase the heart rate and breathing and involve large muscle groups. Some examples are walking/running, cycling outside or on a stationary cycle, cardio machines such as stair-steppers and elliptical trainers, and arms-only cycles. The point is to choose an activity that can be done continuously at a moderate intensity and that is enjoyable.

(continued)

**Designing an Exercise Program to
Improve Health Related Fitness (*continued*)**

■ Muscular strength and endurance are also important
aspects of fitness. There are many ways to incorporate
strengthening exercises into a well rounded program.
These exercises can be performed with weight machines,
free weights, and other modes of resistance such as elastic
bands or even water resistance.

■ Flexibility is another aspect of fitness that should be a
priority. Stretching exercises that focus on the muscles that
have been exercised can easily be added to an exercise
program. In addition, many MS patients have specific areas
in need of stretching due to weakness, spasticity, and
mobility constraints. Flexibility exercises can be used to
maintain or improve range of motion and integrity of joints
and muscles.

AEROBIC EXERCISES

Where you exercise depends on personal tastes as well as physical
capabilities. Some people thrive in structured environments and enjoy
the atmosphere where other people are exercising with them. Group
classes based in MS programs or health clubs are possible options. The
lure of the outdoors and nature are motivational for many people who
enjoy walking in natural areas or parks near home. Other people have
access to and enjoy water-based exercise, either swimming or some type
of aqua exercise. In deciding on an exercise mode, personal preferences
should be considered:

■ Walking/running

■ Exercise ergometers: arm/leg cycles, steppers, elliptical trainers

■ Resistance balls

■ Water Exercise—swimming, water aerobics

In addition to personal preferences, it is important to consider a type of exercise that is compatible with abilities. As mentioned earlier, MS symptoms such as weakness, fatigue, or balance difficulties can impair certain abilities. For individuals with these challenges, weight-supported exercises such as stationary cycling, rowing, and aqua exercise are recommended. For some people with MS, limitations in strength and mobility may require supervision.

MUSCULAR STRENGTH AND FLEXIBILITY EXERCISES

Some types of exercise that are used mainly for aerobic benefits can also be utilized to improve muscular strength. For example, an aquatics exercise class typically devotes a period of time to strengthening exercises, performed with water as resistance. If a health club is where an individual chooses to perform aerobic exercise, the weight machines or free weight equipment can be used for strengthening. There are many exercises designed to improve muscular strength and endurance. Before undertaking such a program, a consultation with a professional is recommended, as proper technique is essential. A physical therapist, exercise physiologist, or certified strength trainer can be very useful in assessing which type of strength exercises would be most beneficial. If exercises with weights are not appealing, there are other ways to improve strength. Pilates is an excellent form of exercise that can be used to strengthen core muscles, as well as the upper and lower extremities. In addition to strength benefits, Pilates also improves flexibility, and classes can be modified to accommodate many of the limitations that people with MS may have. Other forms of exercise such as yoga and Tai Chi can be very useful to people with MS. Although they may not provide aerobic benefits, they are excellent for improving flexibility and even balance. Plus, the meditative aspects of these exercise forms are very appealing to many people.

EXERCISE INTENSITY

Once an exercise type is selected, the next decision becomes the intensity of that exercise. Many people feel that if they are not suffering while they exercise, then it is not working. This idea of "no pain, no gain" may be utilized for athletes preparing for an athletic event, but it is certainly not relevant to health-related fitness. Health benefits result from regular physical activity that is "moderate" in intensity. So, how does one know what moderate is?

Exercise intensity should be monitored subjectively using effort rather than heart rate as the indicator. The Rating of Perceived Exertion (RPE) scale can be used to gauge this effort.

Rate of Perceived Exertion

0   Nothing

1   Very, Very Light

2   Very Light

3   Moderate

4   Somewhat Hard

5   Hard

6

7   Very Hard

8

9   Very, Very Hard

10 Maximal

For cardiovascular health, "moderate" aerobic activity is recommended. The exercise intensity that feels "moderate" to an individual depends on fitness and functional levels. For example, a person who has not been physically active at all might be able to comfortably do about 10 minutes of moderate aerobic exercise. If 10 minutes seems too long, it is probably because the intensity is too high. For those just getting back to a more active lifestyle, it is better to exercise at too easy a level rather than pushing too hard. Most people can exercise at an intensity of "hard" or "very hard" for at least a minute or two, longer if they are physically fit. However, there is no need to work at that level for health benefits—moderate is sufficient.

One reason so few people exercise on a regular basis may be because they tend to work at too high an intensity. In our immediate-results-oriented culture, many people try to make up for years of inactivity by attempting a program that is too ambitious, hoping for quick and drastic results. Although it may be possible to exercise for 30 minutes or more at intensities above "moderate," the payback is often disheartening. Muscle soreness, fatigue, and even injuries can result. A more reasonable approach is to add exercise into the routine gradually and in a way that is pleasurable. Although the end results of an active lifestyle—improved fitness, healthier cardiovascular system, and so on—are worthy goals, the *process* should by enjoyed. Thus, choosing an activity that is fun instead of dreading the next workout will create enthusiasm. At the very least, the goal is to feel better afterwards.

The unpredictable course of MS as well as daily fluctuations in fatigue and energy can make planning physical activity more tricky. Many symptoms of MS, especially fatigue, may interfere with the level of physical activity that is possible on a particular day. This is when the use of the RPE scale is very useful. The RPE scale allows for flexibility that is necessary when MS symptoms are in play. By using effort perception as a guide, physical activities can be adapted to fit the day's functional and energy levels, rather than giving up on physical activity all together. The key is to adjust exercise intensity and duration as MS symptoms fluctuate. One day "moderate" might mean a brisk walk; on another day "moderate" could mean a walk at a much slower pace and for a shorter distance.

Intensity of strength and flexibility training can also be monitored using the RPE scale. When lifting weights or exercising against resistance, the effort should be moderate. Muscles adapt to stresses that are beyond usual loads, but the stress should not be too great. Because soreness and injury can result from loads that are too heavy, it is best to gradually increase resistance over time. With respect to flexibility, stretches should be performed to the point of tension and not pain. Over time the effects of both of these forms of exercise will be realized.

At the beginning of a new exercise program, people normally feel tired after a workout but usually feel back to normal an hour or two afterwards. If exercise produced exhaustion the next day, it may have been too intense and the next workout should be at a lower intensity. Additionally, exercise can be manipulated in duration either by dividing the time into shorter periods or by shortening the entire duration. Instead of exercising for 30 minutes at one time, divide the task into several 5 to 10 minute periods.

EXERCISE DURATION AND FREQUENCY

For health benefits, aerobic exercise should be performed for about 30 minutes, 3 to 5 days per week. A non-exerciser cannot realistically jump to this goal. When just beginning, consistency should be a primary goal. This means showing up on the 3 days and performing the program, even if the duration and intensity are very low to start. With adaptation to the routine and the exercises, duration and intensity can be increased. A more reasonable approach would be to set aside a period of time 3 days per week and start with shorter sessions.

Example of Exercise Duration and Intensity ★

Monday	2-3 Minute warm up—light intensity
	10 Minutes—Moderate intensity
	2-3 Minute cool down—light intensity
Tuesday	Strengthening Exercises
	5 Minutes—stretching
Wednesday	2-3 Minute warm up—light intensity
	10 Minutes—Moderate intensity
	2-3 Minute cool down—light intensity
Thursday	Strengthening Exercises
	5 Minutes—stretching
Friday	2-3 Minute warm up—light intensity
	10 Minutes—Moderate intensity
	2-3 Minute cool down—light intensity

A good rule of thumb is to keep the rate of progression to about 10 percent per week. Thus, if the weekly duration is 30 minutes for the aerobic portion of a program, increase it only by 3 minutes total for the next week. Keeping an exercise diary is a good way to plan your workouts and provides feedback with respect to progress.

Duration for strength exercises works a little differently. The number of exercises being done will likely stay fairly constant, so the time it takes to do a workout will stay the same over time. What will change is the amount of resistance for each exercise. If biceps curls are part of the program, lifting 10 pounds may be a start with being able to comfortably complete 10 repetitions. After doing all of the exercises in the routine (probably about 6–10 exercises), repeating them again will complete the work out. This means completion of 2 sets. As time goes by, 10 pounds for biceps curls will start to get easier. When this happens, the number of repetitions can be increased. Once the repetitions are up to 15, it is time to increase the weight. If the weight is now 12 pounds, the repetitions may go back to about 8 to 10. All of the weight training exercises in this routine can be progressed in this manner. If stretch bands are used, resistance can be altered by changing the length and/or thickness of the bands.

WHAT CAN I DO?

Instead of looking for a magic silver bullet to conquer fatigue, a combination of small, common sense ideas can extend your energy throughout the day. It works!

FATIGUE

Special Considerations for Exercise and MS: Suggestions From an Occupational Therapist

MS fatigue is more than "normal" fatigue. This symptom affects 80 percent to 90 percent of people diagnosed, and a majority of people feel it is the most debilitating aspect of MS. When fatigue is a constant presence, it can be overwhelming. Although it is known that exercise is an important component of maintaining and improving health, the idea of integrating an exercise program in the face of fatigue can be daunting.

One important component of rehabilitation is teaching individuals with MS energy management strategies to counteract symptoms of fatigue. The goal of these strategies is to make daily activities more efficient by modifying, simplifying, and adapting them, to gradually increase energy and independence. The use of these strategies will help implement and maintain an exercise program and keep it going.

A good beginning strategy is to take a personal inventory of energy levels. For this inventory, think of "gaining energy," not "fighting fatigue." This thought alone triggers energy. Next, keep a daily activity log for 5 to 7 days. Write down every activity performed and note the level of energy expended for each activity. Energy levels can be recorded by using a number system. For instance, use a scale of 1 to 10, with "1" meaning extremely low energy, and "10" meaning extremely high energy. During the day, look for patterns of high and low periods of energy. Most people find that a pattern does exist. With this knowledge, activities and exercise can be planned accordingly. An exercise program should be prioritized and scheduled during the period of day when the most energy exists. A number scale can help identify what number represents "good energy." For example, a "7," could mean "good" energy. This, then, is a good time to schedule exercise.

Organizing and plugging exercise into a time slot will improve your follow through and success. As suggested by Dr. Engstrom, people are more successful in completing a task if it is scheduled at a given time. Otherwise, it might be just an idea floating through the day. Tasks should be small and simple. If a routine is gradual and achievable, then exercise will more naturally flow into a daily ritual.

Always pace exercise. If planned and scheduled exercise cannot be completed as intended, stop and acknowledge that some benefit has been achieved. Too often people give up because they feel that if they don't meet their expectations, they have failed. Re-examine the expectations that have been set and determine if they are too high or consider if they are too low.

Integrating an exercise program is not that difficult to do. However, when fatigue is a daily challenge, it may stifle your attempts to exercise. Take small steps in changing how and when activities are performed. Be aware of how energy develops and fatigue lessens when exercise and energy management become a regular routine.

WHAT CAN I DO?

Remember to resist procrastination and let go of guilt. All guilt does is drain energy!

BEAT THE HEAT!

Suggestions From the Exercise Physiologist

Exercise Environment. Creating and adapting an exercise program requires thinking about the environment where it is being performed. Many individuals with MS are heat sensitive, meaning they experience temporary symptom worsening with increases in body temperature. When temperature increases, nerve conduction is affected. In healthy, myelinated nerves, increased temperature increases conduction speed, but in nerves that have some demyelination this increased rate of transmission can be a problem. When current moves across a poorly myelinated area of a nerve, there is "leakage" which results in conduction slowing or sometimes even conduction block. Thus, the message carried by the nerve arrives later or not at all. If the message happens to be to "move the leg," it may not be able to be done as efficiently, or at all, if there is overheating.

Suggestions From the Physical Therapist

A cool pool is a wonderful way to obtain exercise and it can help lower the core body temperature. This will help with feeling better and will assist with overall physical function. The pool can be used by swimmers and non-swimmers alike. Lap swimming is excellent for cardiovascular fitness, but aquatic exercises can also be beneficial. The resistance of moving through water is good for strengthening. Equipment such as Styrofoam dumbbells, hand paddles, noodles, and jogging or buoyancy vests are also useful. A buoyancy vest can keep a person upright to allow them to walk or jog in deep water. Balance is also nicely challenged in the water. Water can also help decrease swelling in the legs. Someone who experiences difficulty with mobility on land may find great freedom of movement in the water. One person with MS said that they wished they could live their daily life in three feet of water! This was someone who could not walk on land, but was free to do so in the pool.

Suggestions From the Occupational Therapist

If heat sensitivity is an issue, there are a number of ways to control the environment. Cooling devices such as vests or even a cool, wet bandana around the neck can be helpful. Exercise performed indoors with air conditioning or fans is also a good option, as is outdoor exercise during the cooler times of day. Evaporative cooling can be increased by spraying water during exercise. Precooling is another simple option and can be done by sitting in a bath filled with cool (not icy) water. Twenty minutes of precooling can deep cool the muscles of the legs and keep the body cool for several hours, depending on how much activity is performed and how hot the day is. It is also important to drink enough fluids so that the ability to dissipate heat through sweating is maximized. If heat is an issue during exercise and there is a change in symptoms, cooling off afterwards should return function to baseline.

If the opposite exists, and sensitivity to cold is an issue, consider dressing in layers. These layers can be removed as needed. Whether sensitivity to heat or cold exists, an exercising person should wear light weight, loose fitting clothes.

Safety Issues in the Exercise Environment

Another environmental factor is lighting. If a room is poorly lighted, it may place more demands on both the visual and balance systems. Natural sunlight is the best source of light.

If exercise equipment is used, it should be adjusted by a trained professional to fit the person using it, thus avoiding inefficient mechanics and wasted expenditures of energy. If needed, adaptive devices can be used to make specific exercises attainable and successful. Many types of stationary and road bikes exist. Both aerobic and yoga classes can be performed while seated with "props" to adapt. Also, walking sticks are popular for assisting balance. It is safe to say that for almost any exercise, there is a way to modify and adapt it. You can check with National MS Society chapters to find local exercise classes, or discuss with your provider and request a referral to a physical or occupational therapist.

WHEN MS SYMPTOMS INTERFERE WITH YOUR ABILITY TO BE PHYSICALLY ACTIVE

Almost all persons with MS are able to perform some level of activity. For some, this may be a dramatic step down from what they used to do. For some, they may find themselves being more active than ever before!

For some, MS may be a "wake up call" that forces a person to take a close look at their life and lifestyle. They may make changes that have been needed to be made for a long time. A previous non-exerciser may become fit for the first time in their life. It is ALL RELATIVE! A program can be devised for almost every individual with MS, no matter what their functional level may be.

Overall fitness can be maintained OR improved, even with the diagnosis of MS. This is of paramount importance. Being unhealthy and unfit is no way to manage MS. If the fitness level is maximized, it will help combat the symptoms of MS.

Just because someone has a diagnosis of MS does not mean that they are exempt from other health risks. Diabetes, heart disease, and cancer are the three main diseases that Americans face. Due to the sedentary lifestyle that we live, people are at a high risk of these diseases even BEFORE the diagnosis of MS. After the diagnosis, that may make it more difficult to find ways to easily and efficiently exercise. But again, there are ways to find this "recipe for success" that will work for each individual. It is known that MS affects each person in a unique way. Sensory problems may inhibit someone from hiking in the woods. Bladder problems may make aquatic exercise a challenge for another individual. Blurred vision may force another person used to outdoor cycling to using a stationary bike.

Where any loss or decline has occurred, it must be determined whether this is reversible or whether acceptable compensations need to be made. This determination should be done by a rehabilitation professional such as a physical therapist.

If a person is fit when the diagnosis of MS occurs, they are more likely to be able to maintain a functional level of health and activity. Of course, if there is a severe exacerbation, recovery to the previous level may be more difficult.

The goal after an exacerbation is to return to a former level of function. A return to baseline may not be possible at first, but it should remain as the goal. An exacerbation may result in the loss of some function without a return to the desired baseline. If this occurs, the status must be re-evaluated and necessary changes and adjustments made.

MS complicates the formula for a healthy lifestyle in several ways. The person with MS is battling a number of compromising factors such as fatigue, weakness, spasticity, problems with balance and coordination, decreased flexibility and range of motion (ROM), and possibly a decreased cardiovascular fitness level and other problems. ALL of these factors must be taken into consideration when devising an individualized program.

SOME DISEASE-SPECIFIC CONSIDERATIONS

Weakness/Spasticity

Muscle weakness is a big problem affecting the ability to exercise in persons with MS. Weakness can be further complicated by an increase in muscle spasticity, or tightness. Conversely, spasticity can actually assist function when it may compensate for certain muscle groups that are very weak. An example would be when spasticity in the legs may allow a person to stand or walk by compensating for extreme muscle weakness. These determinations must be accurately made by the health care professional.

First and foremost, the source of muscle weakness must be identified:

- Is the muscle weak from lack of neurotransmission, where the muscle is just not getting the message from the nerves?

- Is it weak from lack of use due to fatigue?

- Does the person have such problems with balance and coordination that they can't safely perform their current exercise program?

But, if weakness is mainly due to a lack of use or someone being a "couch potato," conventional strengthening exercises will have a great impact. Also, muscle burns more calories than fat, so greater muscle mass can assist with weight loss or maintenance.

There are numerous ways to strengthen muscles. An assessment must be done to determine what types of strengthening are needed and how to best fit this into life. Does this person prefer to work out at home? A gym? With fancy equipment? Indoors? Outside? A number of variables must be explored with the input from the person with MS.

Flexibility/Range of Motion (ROM)

Range of motion can be defined as the movement that a joint or body part has available to move through. Normal ROM can be negatively affected by weakness, spasticity, poor posture, and inactivity because there may be a shortening of muscles secondary to weakness or permanent tightening of soft tissue. It is important to maintain as much ROM throughout the body as possible. This assists in efficient movement, thereby keeping the person as functional as possible.

When ROM or flexibility is compromised, this may have a negative impact on a person's ability to move. This lack of flexibility may also result in pain, such as when the hamstrings or low back muscles are tight low back pain may result. Much time spent in a wheelchair or sitting in general may cause a decrease in ROM in various parts of the body. One can think of how stiff and sore they are when they get out of a car after a long drive.

Again, identifying the area that may be lacking in ROM and identifying the cause of the decreased ROM is paramount in properly treating this problem. A physical therapist is needed for an accurate assessment and to devise a program with positive results.

Flexibility and ROM exercises can be integrated with the rest of the person's fitness program. The pool can augment flexibility/ROM. Balance and coordination activities may enhance ROM. Again, activities that feel good and are enjoyable will prove to be the most successful.

Balance and Coordination

Like the previously mentioned areas, balance and coordination problems can have a variety of causes. The cause must be properly identified to allow for effective treatment. Causes can range from visual disturbances, vestibular problems, weakness, ROM limitations, sensory problems, or medication side effects. Spasticity can also greatly affect balance and coordination. Muscle imbalances can contribute to problems. Is an assistive device needed? If one is being used, is it the proper one for the person's needs, or should it be modified? Is any type of bracing needed? Is fatigue the main contributing factor? Safety is a prime concern where balance and coordination problems exist.

Balance and coordination is another area where overlap can occur with other portions of the person's program. Strengthening can enhance and possibly challenge balance and coordination. Some flexibility activities will definitely have an effect on balance and coordination. Aquatic activities are also useful in improving this area of activity.

Once again, after identifying the cause of lack of balance and coordination and implementing necessary treatment, an exercise routine can be established to meet specific needs.

DESIGNING A THERAPEUTIC EXERCISE PROGRAM

After proper professionals' assessments and clearance from a health care provider to exercise, there are a number of factors to consider. An exercise program should be driven by patient identified priorities. In conjunction with the health care team recommendations, the activities or exercise program should be enjoyable, varied, and realistic. Is the activity accessible? Are the goals attainable? The person with the MS and his or her health care team need to build in accommodations that are sensitive to fluctuations in symptoms. All involved must be aware of barriers such as transportation, time availability, weather, physical assistance needed, equipment required, and other factors that might inhibit the activity from becoming a routine part of the person's daily life.

WHAT CAN I DO?

Develop an exercise program that is individual, enjoyable, and beneficial with the help of professionals such as exercise physiologists, occupational therapists, and physical therapists.

Strengthening

Once the weakness has been identified, explore how to best succeed in this area. A gym? A home program? Free weights? Weight machines? Exercise bands? A DVD to follow? A personal trainer? A supportive support partner? An inflated exercise ball?

In general, a strengthening routine should be done 3 times a week. The area lacking in strength will be the main focus, but overall body strength is equally important. If the lower extremities are weak, make sure the upper extremities stay strong to compensate as needed. If there are respiratory concerns, keeping the chest muscles and postural muscles strong will be important. The physical therapist can help to identify these needs. A variety of exercises will help prevent boredom and overuse injuries. Progression of the program will be monitored by the physical therapist.

Flexibility/ROM

After any areas of tightness or decreased range of motion are identified, ROM activities will need to be incorporated into the exercise program. Will they be stretches that can be done independently? Does the person with MS need to have assistance for certain stretches? Will they be done in a chair, wheelchair, bed, or on the floor? Can a towel, belt, or band/cord assist the movement? These questions need to be addressed by the PT. The more independent the overall program, the better the chance for success.

This is one area of the fitness program that should be done daily. The joints that are limited in range will be the main focus, but overall stretching is needed. It can be done through traditional stretches, yoga, tai chi, stretching in the pool, or with an inflated exercise ball. Maintaining proper muscle length can help alleviate pain and can increase function.

It may be necessary to implement a stretching program to augment the use of assistive devices and/or braces. As previously mentioned, spasticity can assist with function up to a point. The amount of spasticity that is helpful can be assessed by the physician and the PT. Medication may be needed to assist with decreasing spasticity and increasing ROM.

Balance and Coordination

This area also overlaps with the others in an exercise program. Balance, flexibility, and coordination are needed to perform a strengthening program.

Again, the cause of the problems must be accurately identified before treatment is initiated. Treatment can range from medications to resistance ball exercises and balance and coordination activities, including gait training, aquatic activities, yoga, and Tai Chi. An assessment for an assistive device may be important, but proper footwear can make a difference, as can assessing the living and working environments. Shoes may need to be examined by the orthotist, physical therapist, or physiatrist. Flooring may need to be changed. One may need to use a scooter during the work day when traveling long hallways or great distances, thereby saving more energy for exercising or for home activities and obligations. An occupational therapist can greatly assist in this area. Visual disturbances need to be addressed by the appropriate physician. Lighting can also help alleviate some problems with balance and coordination. Safety is of the essence in this area.

CONCLUSION

An exercise program must be one that a person with MS will do. Can Do! The best chances for sticking with the program and achieving success will occur if the program is designed collaboratively with the physical therapist. As previously mentioned, working with a team is important. Make changes in your lifestyle, and then make them again and again and again to accommodate the ever changing nature of MS.

RECOMMENDED READING

Lowenstein, N. (2009). *Fighting Fatigue in Multiple Sclerosis: Practical Ways to Create New Habits and Increase Your Energy.* New York: Demos Medical Publishing.

RECOMMENDED WEBSITES

The National Multiple Sclerosis Society. http://www.nationalmssociety.org
AbleData, Information on Assistive Technology and Assistive Devices for Daily Living. http://www.abledata.com

7 Eating Well, Eating Easy

Baldwin Sanders and Ann Mullinix

Although there are many books about diet and MS, there is no significant scientific evidence that any restrictive diet can change the course of MS. Nevertheless, there are many influences that diet has on health and well-being, and therefore, MS. Diet can be beneficial in alleviating MS symptoms such as fatigue and constipation, and can assist in weight management. Diet can decrease the risk of chronic conditions such as heart disease, cancer, stroke, and diabetes. The U.S. Department of Agriculture and The Department of Health and Human Services have published MyPlate and Dietary Guidelines in an effort to improve America's health and decrease the risk of chronic diseases. A person with MS has the same risk of developing other chronic diseases as anyone else.

A person who eats well feels better and gains all the long term benefits of a complete nutritious diet. A healthy diet does not mean needing to avoid special and enjoyable foods. It is about looking at the overall picture and making choices that provide positive feedback in terms of health and feeling well.

HOW MS AFFECTS DIET

Because the symptoms experienced by those living with the disease are individual, so too are the obstacles to maintaining a healthy diet. Effects of fatigue can be especially difficult to deal with. When fatigued, it is difficult to get the energy to prepare a good meal that provides all the basic food groups. It can interfere with getting a meal on the table. Preparation may be difficult if it requires standing for long periods of time to prepare the ingredients of a recipe. Mobility problems can make it more difficult to do grocery shopping or to move around a kitchen, but skipping meals to avoid the difficulties will only increase fatigue.

The important thing to remember is that small steps can lead to big improvements, and being consistent with the small changes produces results. Contrary to common belief, a healthy diet is one that tastes good. Nutritionists understand that if we are going to convince people to eat better, taste must come into the equation. Also, the less labor intensive to prepare, the more likely people are to eat well.

Understanding that a person's attitude plays a significant role in managing his or her diet is essential. There must be a belief that eating a nourishing diet will benefit overall health. Often, when people start paying attention to what they eat, they find they can enjoy their food more. If well planned, preparation can be an enjoyable and shared activity, making it easier over time. Small, gradual changes will make it easier to accept a new direction in how you eat.

Enlisting the help of others can make food preparation less difficult or tiring. For example:

- Delegate tasks, like washing the vegetables

- Ask family members to help cook dinner and clean up

- Ask for help with shopping

THE EFFECT OF FIBER ON GENERAL HEALTH AND MS

Including more fiber in the diet may increase the life span. In a study published in the *Archives of Internal Medicine*, researchers from the U.S. National Cancer Institute reported that a diet high in fiber may reduce the risk of dying from heart disease, respiratory disease, or any other cause by 22 percent. The average person eats 12 to 15 grams of fiber, while the goal is to consume 25 to 38 grams a day. 25 grams of fiber a day can be obtained with one-third cup of high fiber cereal, a half cup of beans, a small apple with skin, and a half cup of mixed vegetables. Five servings of fruits and vegetables will provide about 15 grams of fiber. Adding ½ cup of beans will add 8 to 10 grams of fiber. Whole grains provide 3 grams per serving.

According to the literature, 50 percent to 68 percent of people with MS have problems with constipation. Because bowel function is a neuromuscular activity, damage to the nerves due to MS results in slowed gastrointestinal motility causing both infrequent and hard stools. Urinary problems may cause decreased liquid intake, which exacerbates constipation. In addition, many of the MS medications have the side effect of constipation. A high fiber diet can be helpful in improving this problem. Many people eat too little fiber, but with MS, this can lead to a significant problem. Getting enough fiber can be achieved by a few additions to the diet such as eating larger amounts of fruits, vegetables, whole grains, and legumes.

WEIGHT MANAGEMENT AND MS

One third of America's population is overweight or obese due to a variety of causes. Due to the decrease in physical activity in some people with MS, caloric requirements are much lower. It is important to be aware of activity levels and calculate portion sizes and calories accordingly.

Weight loss is never the quick or easy process that many advertisements claim. The first goal should be to stop gaining weight and maintain the current weight. Success losing weight can be measured in small dietary changes. Awareness of portion sizes and eliminating drinks and snacks that are high in sugar and calories are examples of small changes. Losing one-half pound per week and keeping it off is real success. Avoid expectations of losing two pounds a week or more as this is almost impossible to keep off and will lead to frustration and a sense of failure. Nourishment, not deprivation, is the goal. Avoid any overly restrictive diets. Losing weight is about learning how to live with a diet that can be sustained and enjoyed over a lifetime. Learn to select your foods carefully and enjoy them more. It is the small steps that lead to success.

One key to managing weight is to eat more fruits and vegetables. Just as the Dietary Guidelines recommend, half of the plate should be fruits and vegetables. These are low calorie foods that are filling and displace large portions of high calorie, high fat foods. Five to nine servings of fruits and vegetables is not unreasonable with the knowledge that one serving equals ½ cup. Add fruit to cereal and yogurt and a variety of breakfast foods. Vegetable soup is a great first course at lunch, and one cup equals two servings. Fruit is a great dessert and snack.

Microwaving double portions of vegetables for dinner can again provide 2 servings, and try cutting up orange or melon slices to put on the plate. Covering a serving of sorbet with strawberries is healthy and easy. In today's world, it is possible to do this with "convenience foods." Grocery stores sell large bags of frozen vegetables and fruits that can make this simple.

Portion sizes in a typical diet have increased. Restaurants fill platters with food, muffins are larger, and an order of French fries continues to grow larger. Portions are four times the size that they were 50 years ago, yet people are far less active.

Looking at the MyPlate recommendations, filling half the plate with fruits and vegetables leaves less room on the plate for meat and starchy foods. Cutting the serving size of meat to 3 or 4 ounces and adding a whole grain food like brown rice will be beneficial. To add dairy to the meal, have frozen yogurt topped with peaches for dessert. Eat slowly and enjoy, and know that a step has been taken toward improving health.

It is important to reduce fats and high fat foods to control weight. Eating smaller portions of meat will help with that. Increasing foods high in fiber can also help to reduce weight because they create a sense of fullness. If hunger is diminished it can help lessen the amount eaten at any meal.

DIET FOR FATIGUE MANAGEMENT

Think of diet as fuel that provides the body with energy. Cars don't run without fuel and neither does the body. Going too long without food pushes hunger and encourages less thoughtful eating. A better option is to eat a snack that takes the edge off hunger, allowing better choices at mealtime. Avoid going longer than 4 to 5 hours during the day without food. A snack should not be more than 200 to 300 calories. It should contain protein, which lasts longer in the system and may increase alertness. A complex carbohydrate is a natural energy food and is utilized more quickly, so when paired with protein, it completes a long lasting, energy producing snack. Mozzarella cheese sticks paired with apples, or crackers are all portable and can be kept in a purse, car, or desk.

Yogurt contains both carbohydrates and protein. Ten to twelve nuts paired with raisins are easy and can be prepared ahead of time. Graham crackers and peanut butter, hummus and wheat crackers, and cottage cheese and fruit make great snacks.

Listen for feedback from the body. Note what works and what doesn't. Try to make meal times and snacks at the same time on a daily basis. If this produces good results, continue. Energy techniques in the kitchen are important as well. Cook in bulk and freeze for later so there will always be a good meal ready to microwave. Soups and casseroles freeze well. When grilling out, grill extra and use it in different dishes.

THE POWER PANTRY

The National MS Society has a great handout, *Food for Thought: MS and Nutrition*, which suggests how to set up a "power pantry." Having healthy foods on hand in the house will allow making good decisions when choosing a meal or a snack and make meal preparation easier. Snacks should contribute to an overall diet and not be something to be indulged in. Make it a habit to keep protein snacks in the refrigerator or in the pantry. Higher calorie or less nutritious snacks are fine, but they should be special and not an everyday occurrence. Be careful not to take care of the lonely, tired, and bored feelings by eating unhealthy snacks. Look for other solutions—read a magazine, water the plants, knit. Make a list for the refrigerator of activities that can provide a detour from mindless eating activities.

CAFFEINE

Caffeine is a stimulant that increases energy, but it has its downfalls as well. Too much caffeine can cause restless sleep and increase fatigue the next day. Some people do use caffeine as a way to manage their fatigue throughout the day, but they are careful about when they utilize it. It is best, for most people, to limit caffeine after noontime. Switching to decaffeinated products in the afternoon may provide the psychological boost without the stimulant. Caffeine also affects bladder function by making it more active. If MS causes bladder symptoms, it is best to limit the use of caffeinated products.

HEALTHY FATS AND MS

In the past, dietary fats have been restricted in many diets by eliminating foods like mayonnaise, butter, and the skin on chicken. An entire industry of low fat and fat free foods was born. The problem with low fat and no fat diets was they were often high in processed carbohydrates and low in complex carbohydrates that are healthier. These processed carbohydrates can lead to elevated triglycerides and blood glucose that can increase the risk of heart disease, stroke, diabetes, hypertension, and diverticulosis.

What is important is eating the right kinds of fat. A large volume of research has been done on the role of fat and heart disease. The American Heart Association has established clear guidelines on the type and amount of fat for Americans to consume. The relationship between dietary fat and MS continues to be examined closely by the scientific community. Studies are preliminary, and there is a need for larger clinical trials, but initial findings indicate that what is good for the heart is good for MS.

Research studies have suggested that polyunsaturated fats, particularly omega-3 fatty acids, have diminished symptoms for relapsing–remitting MS. A two year clinical trial that followed 312 subjects with MS over two years found that the group taking 10 grams of fish oil supplements daily had less disease progression and fewer relapses than those taking a placebo. Other evidence suggests that omega-3 fatty acids exert immunosuppressive actions through their incorporation in immune cells but also may affect cell function within the central nervous system.

Although all fats contain the same amount of calories, those calories are not created equally. Fats can be predominantly monounsaturated, polyunsaturated, and saturated, and always a combination of the three. Monounsaturated and polyunsaturated fats are the "healthy" fats because they can reduce the risk of heart disease. Saturated fats and trans fats are "unhealthy" fats because they increase blood lipids and the risk of heart disease. Good food sources of monounsaturated fats are olive oil and canola oil. Polyunsaturated fats contain omega-3 and omega-6 fatty acids. Omega-3 fatty acids can lower triglycerides and raise HDLs (the good cholesterol), reduce blood clotting, and lower blood pressure. Good food sources of omega-3s are fatty fish such as salmon, mackerel, sardines, anchovies, and tuna. Omega-3s help regulate pro-inflammatory effects of omega-6s, which most Americans get an abundant supply of in their diets. The food industry uses large amounts of soy oil, providing 14 to 25 times more omega-6s in the American diet. The balance between the omega-3 fatty acids and the omega-6 fatty acids is important, so replacing the omega-6 with the omega-3 is beneficial.

The American Heart Association (AHA) and the American Institute of Cancer Research are in agreement regarding fat and health. They recommend a reduction in saturated fats and an increase in omega-3 polyunsaturated fats, and their recommendations are valid for people living with MS as well. Saturated fat and trans fats may raise cholesterol and the risk for heart disease, while omega-3 fatty acids may reduce the risk of heart disease.

The American Heart Association recommends eating two servings of fish every week to provide about 2 grams of omega-3 fatty acids. Many people do not heed this advice. Some don't like fish, others don't know how to prepare it or it is not readily available in their area. Others are concerned about the mercury content of fish. The American Medical Society believes that the benefits of eating fish far outweigh the possible risks of exposure to contaminants. Most fish contain omega-3 fatty acids, but fatty fish, such as salmon, herring, mackerel, lake trout, sardines, and tuna contain larger amounts.

Other sources of omega-3 oils are flaxseed, walnuts, canola oil, and soybean oil. These fats contain alpha-linolenic acid (ALA), which must be converted to omega-3's, and are therefore not as readily available as omega-3's from fish oils.

Fish oils or omega-3 supplements are also an alternative to eating fish. Fish oil contains high concentrations of eicosapentaenoic acid (EPA) and docosahexaenoic acid (DHA). Dosing for fish oil supplements is based on the amount of EPA and DHA rather than the total amount of fish oils. The AHA recommends fish oil supplements of 1 gram daily of EPA and DHA for those with coronary heart disease. Note, however, that supplementing with omega-3 fatty acids increases the body's requirement for Vitamin E, so including a supplement of 100 IU of Vitamin E can protect against a Vitamin E deficiency. Because of the side effects and interactions with medications, it is important to be sure that all health care providers are aware of all supplements taken. Side effects of omega-3 fatty acids include an increased risk of bleeding and may be contraindicated for those taking blood-thinning medications. Omega-3 fatty acids may increase fasting blood sugars and should be used with caution if taking medications to lower blood sugar. The safety of omega-3 supplementation in combination with disease modifying therapies has not been studied, but it is unlikely that these supplements would decrease the effectiveness of the medications.

VITAMIN D AND MS

The link between Vitamin D and MS is a puzzle that has been unfolding for many years. Vitamin D, the "sunshine vitamin," is unique in that it can be obtained from exposure to sunlight as well as from the Vitamin D content of foods. Few foods are good sources of Vitamin D. Milk, fish, and cod liver oil are excellent sources, and more foods are being fortified with extra Vitamin D. The Institute of Medicine (part of the National Academy of Sciences) recently revised the recommended dietary allowance for Vitamin D to be 600 International units (IU) per day for ages 19 to 70 years, and 800 IU per day for people over 70 years of age, with tolerable upper level intakes of 4,000 IU per day. A blood test to evaluate the level of Vitamin D is recommended before supplementation. Vitamin D is an important nutrient for people with MS in two distinctly different ways: Higher levels may prevent osteoporosis and may play a role in decreasing the progression of the disease. For families who have a member with MS (parent, sibling, or child), increasing Vitamin D may reduce the risk of developing MS.

It is well known that Vitamin D is essential for the absorption of calcium and increased bone density. Many factors in MS put people at risk for osteoarthritis, such as frequent treatments with glucocorticosteroids and immobility. It is important that people with MS have strong bones considering their increased risk of falls and fractures.

Recently, scientists have been investigating the possibility that Vitamin D may have an immunomodulatory role in the central nervous system that could benefit people with MS. The potential role of Vitamin D in reducing the inflammatory response and decreasing the severity of disease progression is promising. Active clinical trials are underway to provide evidence of the influence of Vitamin D in MS.

TOOLS FOR PLANNING YOUR DIET

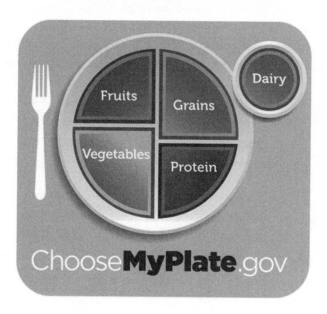

There are several tools that can be used as guidelines for a healthy diet. The newly introduced MyPlate, which takes the place of the USDA Food Guide Pyramid, is not specific to MS but can provide guidelines as to how much of each food group are needed. MyPlate encourages Americans to cover half their plate with fruits and vegetables and the other half of the plate with protein and starch, while encouraging whole grains.

It is easy to go to choosemyplate.gov and enter basic information about age, gender, and physical activity. It will provide a list of nutrient requirements and how much of each food group should be consumed. This can be used as a template to plan a daily diet.

The Dietary Guidelines for Americans are published by the U.S. Department of Agriculture, but the Department of Health and Human Services can also provide guidance relevant to a good diet, at health.gov/DietaryGuidelines. This is the federal government's evidence-based nutrition guidance to promote health, reduce the risk of chronic disease, and reduce the prevalence of overweight and obesity through improved nutrition and physical activity. These guidelines are just as important for those with MS as they are for the wider population. The guidelines are based on the latest scientific information and are more generalized strategies than MyPlate. The emphasis is to encourage the consumption of more vegetables, fruits, whole grains, fat-free or low-fat dairy products and seafood. It is also important to decrease the intake of sodium, saturated and trans-fats, added sugars, and refined grains. Because two-thirds of adult Americans are overweight or obese, the most recent guidelines promote caloric moderation.

Ways to Eliminate Extra Calories

■ Avoid mindless eating where one is not paying attention to the food they are eating and not truly enjoying it.

■ Avoid carelessly eating at a restaurant where portion sizes are the same for a football player as for an older woman.

■ Avoid overindulging in snacks. Snacks should contribute to our diets, restore energy, and prevent fatigue.

Another recommendation from the guidelines is to drink water rather than high sugar drinks such as soft drinks. A twelve ounce can of soda provides approximately 150 calories but does not increase the sense of fullness.

Incorporating these guidelines into everyday lives can improve overall health and well-being. The key guidelines are simple and critical to health. Finding easy ways to incorporate them into a lifestyle will enhance the diet without producing a feeling of having to give up favorite foods.

Key Recommendations of the 2010 Dietary Guidelines for Americans

■ Enjoy food, but eat less

■ Avoid oversized portions

■ Make half the plate fruits and vegetables

■ Switch to fat-free or low-fat milk

(continued)

Key Recommendations of the 2010 Dietary Guidelines for Americans (*continued*)

- Compare sodium in foods like soup, bread, and frozen meals, and choose the foods with the lower numbers
- Drink water instead of high sugar drinks

A DIET FOR MS

- A diet for MS is one that decreases the risk of chronic disease, as recommended by the Dietary Guidelines and the MyPlate food guide for all Americans. It is high in omega-3 fatty acids, as is recommended by the American Heart Association. It is high in fiber. It is planned so that snacks will decrease fatigue and improve energy levels. It takes into account fatigue that may interfere with the preparation of food, as well as the expense of eating well.

- Breakfast is a good meal to consume protein, fiber, and fruit. Try a high fiber cereal that has at least 5 grams of fiber per serving. For lower fiber cereals, add a tablespoon of a high fiber cereal such as Fiber One or All Bran. Gradually increase the high fiber cereal to 2 to 3 tablespoons. These cereals can also be added to yogurt for a snack. Adding a banana to a bowl of cereal can boost fruit intake. Skim milk will provide protein. Breakfast burritos with eggs, low fat cheese, and leftover potatoes and onions can be frozen and reheated for a quick breakfast. Oatmeal with added dried fruit is a nutritious choice for cold mornings. Toast and peanut butter can supply long lasting energy.

- For lunch, soup and a salad, a sandwich on whole grain bread or a wrap, or black beans and rice with coleslaw and a corn muffin are good choices. Fruit, fresh or frozen, completes the nutrition value.

- For dinner, grilled chicken (with extra to make fajitas for another meal), vegetables, and a baked sweet potato is a filling and healthy meal.

- Food intake can be a significant part of a family's budget. A diet needs to taste good and be affordable. Eating out at restaurants is an easy solution to fatigue, but with the average American eating 4.2 meals

113

out per week, it is an expensive solution. Eating out at restaurants often leads to over-indulgence in calories, fats, and other non-nutrients. Eating at home should be as pleasurable as it is to eat out.

WHAT CAN I DO?

Here are some examples of small steps you can take to improve your diet. Try a few at a time. Refer to the chapter on goal setting and include these suggestions.

- Make a big pot of soup and freeze in individual servings for later.

- Add a piece of fruit for dessert at lunch.

- Double up on your vegetables at dinner.

- Start your morning with a high fiber cereal topped with bananas or other fruit.

- Grilling Out? Grill twice the amount of chicken and use later in various ways—on top of a salad, diced into spaghetti, or to make fajitas.

- Keep a fruit bowl on your desk, rather than a candy dish. Evidence shows that you are much more likely to consume either if they are on your desk.

- Try bulgur or quinoa recipes for supper. There are plentiful recipes on the Internet.

- Eat more beans. Bean burritos, bean soups, beans and rice, and bean chili are examples.

- Include small protein based snacks in your diet to take the edge off your hunger.

- Try a fruit smoothie for breakfast using yogurt and frozen fruit.

GETTING IT TO YOUR TABLE

Occupational therapists recommend simplifying the meal process. Having the desire and motivation to eat well is one thing, but the process of actually carrying it out, from purchasing the food to placing a meal on the table, is another. Obstacles are real, such as limited time and energy, or challenges from cognitive and physical changes. People too often feel defeated before meal preparation even begins. Being flexible, open to change, and having a positive attitude can make healthy eating achievable. Implementing a few simple strategies will help in "getting it to the table."

■ First and foremost, be realistic. Keep meals simple. Plan meals 3 to 5 days in advance. Create a menu and write it down, which helps keep accountability. Make a grocery list of all the food items or ingredients that are needed and take advantage of pre-washed and pre-cut foods. Organize a grocery list by how food is grouped at the store, such as dry items, meats, produce, dairy, and bakery. This way, healthy choices are more likely to be made and energy saved. Try new recipes when there is optimal time and energy available. Eating well may mean adding more vegetables to a pasta dish, or having frozen fruits on hand for a smoothie. Think of small changes and build upon them.

■ Plan grocery shopping during a period of good energy, and avoid heavy traffic times at the store. Also, ask some questions. Are there any alternatives to shopping? Should this task be delegated? Since there is a thorough list, should the groceries be ordered on-line and delivered? Should a scooter be used to save energy and direct attention and concentration on the task of shopping instead of on balance? At the check-out counter, request to pack similar items together, such as items that are frozen, items that need refrigeration, or items that are stored in the pantry. Keep bags light. This process will simplify putting items away at home.

■ While putting groceries away, think if there are better places to store food. Frequently used items should be in convenient, easy-to-reach places. Get rid of clutter! If it's hard to reach around a serving platter only used occasionally, store it in a different location. If it hasn't been used in a year, get rid of it permanently! Use a cart with wheels instead of carrying items, or use a stool with wheels to sit on while moving items.

■ Sitting to prepare meals saves energy, strength, and balance. At the start of food preparation, obtain the items needed to make a meal: ingredients, cooking utensils, and any equipment. This will save time and eliminate the need to move back and forth.

- The kitchen environment can influence the success of cooking. Be aware of the temperature of the room. Is it too warm? Check the lighting. Is it too bright? Are there distractions that need to be dealt with? Sometimes these background factors generate more stress on our minds and bodies than we realize.

- Meal preparation can be simplified by using electrical appliances such as mixers, grills, food processors, and can/jar openers. Built up handles on utensils, and suction cups under bowls and cutting boards make them easier to hold and stabilize. One-handed rocker knives come in all sizes. Enlarged stove knobs and color-coded measuring cups are helpful to compensate for blurry or low vision. These are just some examples of adaptive devices used to make tasks easier if physical functions, such as strength or coordination, have changed. Visit websites, request a catalog, or go to any medical supply company to learn more about the various adaptive equipment products available.

- A good idea when preparing meals is to think ahead. Double the recipe and freeze half for another day. In addition to the extra frozen turkey chili made the night before, keep potential meal ingredients on hand for a stand-by nutritious meal. Pacing and preparing parts of a meal a few days ahead, especially if preparing food for a dinner party, decreases stress and makes the meal feel doable.

- Oh, yes, then there is always the clean-up. Make choices about where to spend energy. If preparing a meal is the goal and cleaning is not of interest, compromise: Use disposable plates; soak pots, pans, and dishes overnight; sit on a stool to wash dishes or place them in a dishwasher. And always, stay cool and hydrated.

Dr. Dave Engstrom speaks about removing barriers to achieve goals. Do away with any possible barriers that come from the mind. This encourages being positive and flexible. When willing to work within a schedule and set limits, it will allow for imperfections and compromise. Do away with external barriers and make the environment accessible to meet needs and encourage support from family or friends. Remember, sharing a meal together is about fellowship. Make mealtime a positive experience and know that healthy eating can be done with a few common sense changes and an open mindset.

RECOMMENDED READING

Adelson, R. (2011). "Symptom Management Highlight: Bowel Issues." *Momentum* 4: 38–41.

Bowling, A., and T. Stewart. (2010). *Vitamins, Minerals & Herbs in MS: An Introduction*. Washington, DC: National MS Society.

Mark, B. L., and J. S. Carson. (2006). "Vitamin D and Autoimmune Disease-Implications for Practice from the Multiple Sclerosis Literature." *Journal of American Dietetic Association 106*: 418–24.

Nowack, D. (2008). *Food for Thought: MS and Nutrition*. Washington, DC: National MS Society.

Schwarz, S. P. (2006). *Multiple Sclerosis: 300 Tips for Making Life Easier*. 2nd ed. New York: Demos Medical Publishing.

Vitamin D: Hope on the Horizon for MS Prevention? (2010). The Leading Edge. *Lancet Neurology* 9: 555.

RECOMMENDED WEBSITES

The National Multiple Sclerosis Society. http://www.nationalmssociety.org

AbleData, Information on assistive technology and assistive devices for daily living. http://www.abledata.com

8 Caring for Total Health

Patricia Kennedy

I'm not sitting here languishing, waiting for a cure. I am dedicated to maintaining my overall health because it helps me live the best life possible.

Jimmie Heuga

Learning how to live a full life in the face of a chronic disease such as MS means that one must look beyond the diagnosis. A person with MS continues to be a whole person who needs to attend to maintaining good health and who needs to interact with the world around them through lifestyle changes, improved interpersonal interactions, and feeling empowered to improve quality of life and exploration of one's inner strengths. Just as someone who isn't dealing with illness still faces traumas and dilemmas, a person with MS does also. Both need to be managed to move on.

"Just because you have a chronic illness doesn't mean you have to be chronically ill" is a comment from many people living with MS. Health is a continuum through life. When illness—either acute or chronic—occurs, it is typical for people to make attempts to return to health. Although challenging at times, reaching that state of health provides a sense of achievement and satisfaction. In the case of a chronic condition, people report that same satisfaction in achieving a subjective state of good health.

It is not uncommon for people with MS to feel overwhelmed by it. Other issues such as attending to health in general, strengthening their support systems, engaging in activities such as exercise, or indulging in leisure activities can become secondary. It is also hard to recognize inner skills of resiliency or deep-seated spirituality. To reinstate balance and to move forward, address the issues that are in need of attention.

In general, overall health is a concern for all. More people die annually from conditions that are considered "non-communicable diseases" than any other cause. The big ones include heart conditions, cancer, chronic lung diseases, and diabetes. But others such as kidney failure, cirrhosis, and arthritis are growing as well. This means that preventable conditions are being ignored by the general public. This also means that you have a greater chance of dying of one of these diseases than you do from multiple sclerosis.

These Non-Communicable Diseases are Fueled by Behavior Such as Smoking, Obesity, Inactivity, and Alcohol Consumption

- Cardiovascular diseases
- Cancer
- Chronic lung disease
- Diabetes
- Kidney failure
- Arthritis
- Cirrhosis

One needs only to look at statistics to see the impact of poor health behavior and lifestyle changes.

- 63 percent of deaths worldwide are related to these diseases
- Men and women are affected equally
- 6 million people die yearly from the consequences of tobacco use
- 3.4 million people died from consequences of elevated blood sugar in 2004
- 1.5 billion adults were overweight in 2008

This book addresses nutrition, exercise, relationships, personal strengths, working with a team to achieve good MS care, and managing MS from a team perspective. In addition, it is important to look at ways to address lifestyle changes, take steps to attend to total health, and evaluate inner strengths.

Stepping away from MS management to view these other issues may feel like a challenge. It may feel that there are too many disjointed problems. Deciding which area to address first can be overwhelming.

Caring for total health, lifestyle issues, and personal inner strengths are a part of the whole, even though they feel like unrelated issues when evaluated separately.

Our health care system feeds this concept of separation between body, mind, and spirit. The days of receiving all health care in one location are gone. Now, we talk about teams. It takes more effort to find the care and resources we need. When contemplating making lifestyle changes, no one person has all the answers. The American Medical Association is making a concerted effort to educate its members to identify lifestyle issues as a primary concern and then to discuss these issues with their patients. They are also stressing the importance of knowing where resources are in individual communities and referring patients and families to them. In addition, they strongly encourage their members to personally take better care of their own health through lifestyle changes in order to serve as an example to the community.

Resiliency and spirituality, as a part of our personal health, are important aspects of total health. For many, they are the glue that holds it all together. Attention to these subjects is part of what allows a person with a chronic disease to achieve that sense of subjective well being.

WHERE TO START?

If dealing with MS, the assumption is made that most people have established care with a neurologist. For some, that physician becomes the sole care provider for them as MS takes up so much of their medical attention. However, neurologists are not primary health care providers; they are specialists in neurologic illnesses. Primary care providers are usually specialists in family practice or internal medicine, and people with MS need to be in the care of one of them. Initially, it may be difficult to know which symptoms are related to MS and which are not. If problems arise, contact the provider that might seem the most logical. If another provider is thought to be more appropriate, ask for the reasons for that decision. It is not uncommon for busy providers to view a person living with MS through blinders, ignoring the other potential causes of symptoms. As a health care team is established, encourage (or insist) that both the neurologic provider and the primary care provider are mindful of all health care issues and communicate with each other. Plan to see the primary provider on a regular basis. Be sure to inform that provider of MS treatments being utilized, including medications and rehabilitative measures. If complementary treatments are being used, keep the providers aware.

Establishing a working relationship with providers is a part of improving health. As Dr. Randall Schapiro says, "MS is a marathon, not a sprint." Find time to work on these relationships. It will often take several visits to feel comfortable in that relationship. A recent survey of primary providers found that forming a relationship is the most important thing a patient can do for better health care. The relationship should be a two way street. People who respect and partner with their physicians are more apt to feel in control of their health, tolerate treatments better, and will take more responsibility for maintaining and promoting their health.

Routine and Preventative Care

Be knowledgeable of all routine and preventative recommendations throughout a life span. Become aware of recommendations for routine care based on age, gender, ethnicity, and family and personal history. A resource for these recommendations appears at the end of this chapter. Some of these recommendations include:

- Pap tests for women
- Breast and testicle exams
- Rectal examinations
- Mammograms
- Colonoscopies
- Routine blood tests for lipids, thyroid function, complete blood count, and blood chemistry

(continued)

Routine and Preventative Care (*continued*)

- Bone density studies
- Prostate examinations and blood tests

LIFESTYLE CHANGES

If you change the way you look at things, the things you look at change.

Dr. Wayne Dyer

Earlier in this chapter, a list of serious health problems was mentioned. While some of these issues are discussed in other chapters, there are additional ones to mention here:

- Smoking
- Excessive or frequent alcohol use
- Dental health
- Weight management
- Sleep
- General recommendations

Smoking

For many health reasons, it is recommended for all people to stop smoking or to not start smoking. For people with MS, it is even more important to follow that advice. People with relapsing/remitting MS who smoke are more likely to transition to secondary progressive MS sooner. Family members such as parents, siblings, or children who smoke have a greater risk of developing MS. Secondary smoke has similar effects.

Alcohol

Alcohol affects cognition, walking, and balance in anyone. It can potentially increase those problems already existing in a person with MS.

In addition, alcohol can increase depression as well as reduce quality of sleep. While alcohol may seem, initially, to be a stress reducer, other management tools may be more beneficial in the long run.

Dental Health

Poor dental hygiene can cause a person to feel unhealthy in general and can lead to infections of the gums and teeth. For someone with MS, this may impact the disease and its symptoms as any infection might. If a wheelchair is needed, ask the dental office staff in advance if the office and equipment are accessible.

Sleep

Maintaining healthy sleep is important, as sleep disorders are associated with an increased risk of mortality, cardiac disease, obesity, stroke, and diabetes. Sleep disorders are more common in people with MS. They also can contribute to depression, pain, and fatigue.

 Sleep Problems Occur for Many Reasons

- Sleep apnea
- Insomnia
- Circadian rhythm disorder
- Restless legs syndrome
- Spasticity
- Pain
- Inability to move freely in bed
- Bladder frequency

While these issues should be discussed with the primary provider or neurology provider, there are measures an individual can do on her or his own.

- Sleep Hygiene
  - Maintain a sleep schedule
  - Avoid napping more than one hour

- Avoid alcohol and caffeine before bed
- Avoid a heavy meal before bed time
- Exercise regularly but not before sleep

■ Getting Ready For Bed
  - Have a light snack
  - Limit liquid intake one hour before bed time
  - Do relaxation techniques
  - Clear the mind
  - Establish a consistent sleep ritual

■ Sleep Environment
  - Do not spend the daytime in the bedroom
  - Maintain a comfortable temperature
  - Assure comfortable bedding
  - Eliminate sources of light
  - Do not watch TV in the bedroom
  - Reserve the bed for sex and sleep only

General Recommendations

■ Always wear a seatbelt: in a car, in a wheelchair, on a ski lift, or on a roller coaster.

■ Always wear a helmet when cycling, climbing, skiing, boarding, or zip lining. A brain is a terrible thing to waste!

■ Avoid excessive sun exposure. Although some exposure to sunshine is beneficial, too much exposure damages skin and increases the risk of skin cancer.

■ Request an assessment of total body skin yearly to identify skin cancer early.

PERSONAL STRENGTH

When diagnosed with a chronic disease such as MS, feelings of loss of control and loss of self efficacy often occur. Self efficacy is a person's belief in his or her ability to succeed in a particular situation. This can be accompanied by a loss of self empowerment. By taking charge of overall health, one begins to feel control over many aspects of life including MS. Succeeding at making positive changes improves self efficacy or the feeling of "I can do this!" which leads to more successes over time. Asking questions, seeking resources, asking for help, and forming a team will enhance a sense of empowerment in all aspects of health. Empowerment opens many doors as an individual and as a member of the community at large. Imagine the boost in self esteem when goals are reached and barriers diminish. That power can serve as a spark to do more, either individually or for someone else who needs help. Many of our best volunteers are people who have been empowered to share their talents and time.

RESILIENCE AND SPIRITUALITY

As people with MS are able to feel more in control of their disease and all the issues involved with it, it is appropriate that they move forward to become individuals who have MS but also have other equally important parts to their lives. Getting to that place takes coping skills, resilience, and time. It is not a smooth road. It comes with mixed emotions, fear, feelings of isolation, and questions of the presence of purpose in life.

Resilience

In life, most people face crises. Each one helps form coping skills. Reflect back on how these skills have worked before—some may be helpful now. People are resilient. This is defined as an ability to recover from or adjust easily to misfortune or change. Resiliency also means the ability to "bounce back" or "break through" instead of breaking down. Resilience helps people feel optimistic and persevering. It helps build inner strength allowing people to handle uncomfortable feelings and to be able to think clearly and logically under pressure.

Attending to Spiritual Health

Spirituality means different things to different people. It is not necessarily a religion. It can be a component or extension of our emotional and mental health. Spiritual health helps develop life purpose, allows trust, and helps us let go of those things that are not controllable. It fosters acceptance of situations and our personal being, giving the ability to move forward. It allows forgiveness. Strengthening this part of health may promote emotional healing and offer hope of something better. Inner strength and beliefs are continuously developing and changing but need to be nourished, actively worked on, and allowed time of their own.

Spirituality is unique to each individual and is an intentional journey. Some examples of those journeys are:

- Devotions

- Meditations

- Reading

- Mind/body practices such as yoga

- Quiet and solitude of being alone and listening

These inner strengths and journeys increase simplicity of life, appreciation of natural beauty, and enjoyment of daily experiences with the goal of increasing awareness of positives in life and not focusing on the negatives. The interpretation of these can change with the seeking and acknowledgment of a greater power.

RECOMMENDED WEBSITE

Selected Preventative Screening Recommendations:
http://www.cdc.gov/nccdphp/dnpao/hwi/resources/preventative_screening.htm

9 Support Partners

Rosalind Kalb

Put on your own oxygen mask before assisting the person next to you.

That message, which is heard at the beginning of every airplane trip, is also important for support partners embarking on the MS journey. In order to provide care and support for a loved one—whether the person is a spouse, partner, child, or parent—a support partner must first tend to his or her own health and well-being. For many people who have a loved one with MS, this chapter may be the first time they are being encouraged to pay attention to their own needs. By the end of the chapter, the hope is that support partners will no longer see taking care of themselves as selfish or self-centered, but rather as self-sustaining and self-empowering.

This chapter speaks primarily to support partners who have a spouse or partner with MS. Many of the issues are similar for adult children who have a parent with MS or parents with a child or young adult with MS, but additional resources for them are listed at the end of the chapter.

There is no doubt that when a person is diagnosed with MS, his or her support partner lives with the disease as well. In fact, many couples talk about MS as something they have together. Being a support partner for a person with a chronic, unpredictable disease like MS can be truly gratifying and rewarding. It can also be challenging and draining no matter how much one loves the person or how committed one is to the relationship. For many support partners, the added responsibilities can feel like "a second full-time job" that requires a high level of emotional and physical stamina and leaves no time for leisure or time alone. And most will say that extended family, friends, and colleagues, and even health care providers, have little understanding of the challenges they face. This chapter will take a look at these challenges and provide strategies for managing them more comfortably.

ACKNOWLEDGING THE FEELINGS

The starting point for self-care is acknowledging how one is feeling—both emotionally and physically. Support partners often feel over-whelmed by feelings that have no comfortable outlet:

- **Exhaustion**—The fatigue that comes with a caregiving role can be both emotional and physical. Stress and worry are exhausting, as are the additional responsibilities that seem to fill the hours of the day. Whether or not a person is providing hands-on care, fatigue is a common experience.

- **Sadness and loss**—Just as people with MS need to grieve over changes and losses caused by the disease, support partners do as well. Changes in lifestyle, shared activities, and dreams for the future are some of the losses that support partners experience.

- **Loneliness**—Feelings of loneliness and isolation are common among support partners. They may have no one with whom they can comfortably share their feelings and concerns. Friends and family members may pull away as the MS progresses. Cognitive changes and/or mood issues may make their partner with MS feel "like a different person" or "not like the person I married." And while family, friends, and health care professionals focus their attention on the person with MS, a support partner can begin to feel invisible.

- **Frustration and anger**—Support partners often express frustration or anger at not being able to make things better for the person they love. In spite of their best efforts, the person with MS may continue to decline, to experience great discomfort, to be unable to do things they want to do. Men, in particular, who pride themselves on being able to take charge, handle problems, and fix things, talk about feeling helpless and frustrated. And for support partners who struggle to navigate the health care and insurance maze, access important resources for their partner, or simply keep up with responsibilities at work while trying to manage their support partner role, the feelings of frustration and powerlessness can at times feel overwhelming.

■ **Anxiety**—Anxiety about the future is universal among support partners. The variability and unpredictability of MS make it impossible to know what the future will bring, so worries about progressive disability, financial hardships, and lifestyle changes are common.

Unfortunately, support partners tend to keep the feelings to themselves. When support partners are asked how they are doing, their most common response is "I'm fine—she's/he's the one with MS." As the designated "well person" in the relationship, they have learned to focus on their partner's feelings and well-being to the exclusion of their own:

■ Because support partners are seldom asked by friends, family members, or health care professionals how they are doing or feeling, they can easily come to the conclusion that they're not supposed to have the feelings, let alone talk about them.

■ Since women are at least 2 to 3 times more likely to get MS than men, a significant percentage of support partners are men. And most men in our culture don't talk easily about their feelings even under the best of circumstances.

■ Although women share their feelings more easily, they are somehow expected in our culture to nourish, nurture, and nurse without blinking an eye.

■ Both women and men may keep feelings to themselves because they don't want to worry or upset their loved one with MS.

So for a variety of reasons, the feelings tend to be kept under wraps. The downside is that these feelings can simmer uncomfortably, interfering with a couple's closeness and communication, leading to problems with alcohol or drugs, and even spilling into abusive language or behavior.

MANAGING THE FEELINGS

When given a comfortable opportunity to share feelings with one another, support partners are often astounded and relieved to discover that they aren't alone, that others have similar feelings, and that they can help one another by sharing creative solutions, proactive strategies, and helpful resources, as well as tears and laughter. Many chapters of the National MS Society and other MS advocacy organizations offer self-help groups for support partners. In areas where there are currently no support partner groups, these advocacy groups will help people who would like to start one. Individual counseling, peer counseling with another MS support partner, and online chat rooms for support partners are also excellent options.

WHAT CAN I DO?

How one chooses to connect is less important than making sure one does.

DEALING WITH THE PRACTICAL ISSUES

When support partners begin to talk about their feelings, it becomes clear that much of their stress and anxiety stems from dealing with challenges for which they feel totally unprepared. Whether related to caregiving activities, financial worries, or quality of life issues, they feel at a loss. As they gain more knowledge about MS and available resources and begin to share problem-solving strategies, they feel more prepared and empowered. And with that, comes a sigh of relief and the energy they need to continue providing care and support for their spouse or partner. Following are some practical tips to help support partners feel more prepared:

■ **Providing care**—Support partners express concerns about helping their loved one to remain as healthy, safe, and secure as possible, given the challenges of MS. Unfortunately, the health care team is generally so focused on the needs of the person with MS that they seldom think to provide education and support to the partner, even though the partner is often called upon to participate in the treatment plan. If the doctor or nurse develops a treatment plan that involves the support partner (for example, assistance with injections, exercises, or a catheter), the support partner has a right and a responsibility to ask for guidance, training, and support. And if the treatment plan requires the support partner to do something that is unrealistic or otherwise unacceptable (because of work schedule, other commitments, or strong personal preferences) it is important for the support partner to say so. The treatment plan can't be successful if it is built on unfair or unrealistic assumptions about the support partner's participation.

The Family Medical Leave Act is an important resource for support partners—particularly those who find that they need to take significant amounts of time off to help their spouse or other family member. Simply put, this federal law requires employers in the public and private sectors to hold workers' jobs open and continue paying health insurance premiums while employees take up to 12 (consecutive or non-consecutive) weeks of unpaid leave per calendar year to deal with their own or a family member's serious health condition. The law covers any employer who has 50 or more employees residing within a 75-mile radius of the work location. Employees are eligible for protection under this law if they have worked at the job for at least one year (no fewer than 1,250 hours within the 12 months preceding the requested leave date) and have (or have a family member who has) a serious health condition. The employer must allow the worker to return to the same or a similar, equivalent position unless the employee is a key employee (earning among the highest 10 percent of salaries in the company) or someone whose job cannot be held open without creating substantial and grievous long-term economic injury to the employer's operations.

■ **Managing the finances**—MS is an expensive disease—not only in terms of medical costs but also potential loss of income. It is never too early to start looking at the family's finances in order to ensure financial security in the event that the disease becomes disabling. Too many families shy away from thinking ahead—some because they think it is bad luck or taking too pessimistic a view, and others simply because they find it too scary. However, the simple truth is that support partners can save themselves and their loved one with MS a great deal of stress and anxiety by planning for the worst even while hoping for the best. For most people, the worst doesn't come to pass and MS-related disability doesn't become severe, but planning and preparing for the possibility means that people don't have to spend time and energy feeling anxious about it. In other words, having a financial plan in place is both a financial and an emotional safety net—"If the disease becomes more disabling, we have a financial plan in place to deal with it" is a very comforting thought. People with MS and their support partners can get a free financial planning consultation through the National MS Society's partnership with the Financial Education Partners (FEP) program. Information about this resource is available by calling 800-344-4867. Additional resources are listed at the end of this chapter.

■ **Planning for future care needs**—As with financial planning, it can be both helpful and comforting to plan for future care needs, even if the need never arises. Support partners who have been providing hands-on care for a loved one with more progressive MS have significant concerns about what would happen if they, themselves, were to become ill or die. "Who will take care of him/her if I'm not around?" is a common worry. As with other worries, the best strategy is always to talk with one another about it now and work together to figure out possible solutions. Not only is having a plan reassuring, but it avoids having to make important decisions in the midst of a crisis, when no one is equipped to think clearly or come up with optimal answers. The health care team can be an invaluable resource in these conversations, as can the National MS Society and other MS advocacy organizations. And sharing concerns and ideas with family members can be helpful as well, especially because it helps to avoid tension and conflict in the future.

Support partners are also advised to get their own long-term care insurance. Although the person with MS may not be able to access this kind of insurance after diagnosis, the support partner can be insured against his or her own possible illness or disability.

MAINTAINING QUALITY OF LIFE

MS is an intrusion. For those whose relationship pre-dated the MS, the diagnosis can be compared to having a stranger move into the household and take up residence—definitely a third-wheel that no one wants around. For those whose relationship started after MS was already in the picture, disease progression can make that stranger feel like a bully or a monster. Maintaining one's quality of life in the presence of this kind of intrusion can be very challenging. Some helpful strategies include:

- **Carving out time for oneself is crucial**—"I can't find any time or space for myself" is a common refrain among support partners. They usually whisper it because they feel guilty about wanting and needing it, but they all talk about it. Needing time and space isn't greedy, selfish, or uncaring, it's essential for everyone's well-being.
  - Recreational activities are important to quality of life. When support partners give up activities their loved one can no longer do, the most common results are resentment on the part of the support partner and guilt on the loved one's part. A far better strategy is for each person to engage in at least one activity that they enjoy on their own and for the couple to share familiar activities that they've found a way to adapt for the person with MS, or new activities that both are able to enjoy. Taking time to enjoy a recreational activity or hobby allows a support partner to return refreshed and invigorated.
  - For many support partners, the daily transition from work to home is a critical time. Depending on the kinds of assistance and household responsibilities they handle at home, it can feel like leaving tasks, deadlines, and pressures in one place to pick up another set of tasks, deadlines, and pressures in the other place— in other words, two full-time jobs. And particularly in situations where the person with MS has been home alone without much in the way of activities or companionship, she or he is naturally eager for attention, conversation, and assistance with one thing or another. It is vital for support partners to have some time and space to make the physical and emotional transition. Many report that as little as 15 to 20 minutes can make all the difference—just

a little time to come home, change clothes, and gather their thoughts—before dealing with whatever needs to be done in the way of assistance or household chores.

- Support partners who care for a loved one with significant disability are always on call and always wondering if the person is safe and comfortable. The reality is that these support partners may need to provide assistance of some kind at any time of day or night—and often do. This means that whether awake or asleep they are never able to fully engage in what they're doing because they are always on alert, waiting for whatever the next need or want might be and worrying if everything is okay. They describe it as "wearing an on-call button twenty-four/seven." In these situations, respite options are crucial. Support partners need some periods of time in which they can be fully involved in their own activities.

Respite comes in many forms:

- Knowing that the person with MS is wearing a safety call button in case of falls can relieve the support partner of incessant worries about her or his safety; Inviting a neighbor or friend to visit while the support partner plays an hour of tennis or goes for a hike can make that hour feel worry-free and exhilarating; Having a home health aide come into the home for a few hours each day can allow the support partner to concentrate without worry at work and come home to a household in which some of the chores have already been done.
- Short respite stays in a nursing home facility can make it possible for support partners to go on an important business trip or take a short vacation with the comfort of knowing that their loved one is not alone.
- Working together to identify these options is a way that partners can care for one another, ensuring that each person's needs are met in a healthy and comfortable way.

■ **Getting help**—In the same way that it may take people with MS some time to get comfortable with the idea of asking for help or using a mobility aid, support partners often feel that they should be able to handle everything themselves. In the beginning they may be hesitant to ask others for help or to look for community resources because that would be acknowledging to themselves and others that the challenges are more than they can handle or that the MS is getting worse. Later on they may worry about burdening family and friends, particularly if those people have begun to distance themselves in any way. Being able to access help if and when it's needed is essential for support partners. Not only does assistance from others help ensure optimal care for the person with MS, it also helps prevent the overwhelming feelings of loneliness and isolation that can plague support partners. Assistance can come from family and friends, paid help, or other community resources. The first step is for the support partner and person with MS to talk together about what kinds of assistance would make life more manageable. With that list in hand, they can then figure out how best to get that assistance.

- Family and friends typically want to help but don't know how. The best strategy is for support partners to reach out with specific requests—"When you go to the store, could you please pick up a few things for us?" "Susan has a doctor's appointment on the 13th at 3:00 p.m. and I have a meeting at work that I need to attend. Could you possibly take her?" "Jim has a prescription to be picked up at the pharmacy and I can't leave him right now. Do you think you could get it for me?" "I really need to get out and get some exercise. Would you be able to come by for a couple of hours tomorrow so that I can get to the gym?" It is much easier for people to help when they know exactly what's needed and when.

- Paid helpers can be a huge help even if they only come for a few hours a day or a couple of days a week. Depending on the person's job description and qualifications, she or he may provide companionship, hands-on care, light housekeeping, and other types of assistance. Having a set schedule makes it possible for support partners to plan how to make the best use of that time—whether it's for rest, errands, exercise, or an activity with the children. Paid helpers can be found via home health agencies or through the local grapevine.

- Community agencies and resources can be an invaluable source of help, but most people have no idea what's available. In many areas there are transportation services for the elderly and people with disabilities, grocery stores that will deliver, social service agencies that can provide various types of assistance. Yet, unfortunately, most people wait until there's a crisis of some kind to investigate them. The more effective strategy is to explore the local community *before* there's a crisis. The National MS Society can also help people identify the local resources that are available to them.

■ Making life easier
Life today is complicated for everyone. Families who are dealing with a chronic, unpredictable illness like MS face even greater complexities. The first step to managing the stresses and strains more comfortably is to set priorities. Partners need to negotiate this together since one person's top priority might be very low on the other person's list. By working together, partners can identify activities and tasks that are really important to either or both of them and let the rest go. This helps to ensure that everyone is spending their valuable energy and time on the things that matter most.

•   Another way to make life easier is to optimize the use of technology and other time- and energy-saving strategies to simplify daily routines. Virtually any task can be done the hard way or an easier way, and occupational therapists (OTs) are trained to help people find tools and work-arounds to get things done. Enlisting the skills of the OT provides a dual benefit: the person with MS derives satisfaction from being able to do more things safely and independently, and the support partner is relieved of some chores and able to focus more efficiently on others.

•   The OT can also suggest ways to make the home environment more accessible and user-friendly so that the person with MS can feel productive, safe, and independent. When the home is truly functional, things run more smoothly, everyone feels able to contribute to the household, and worries about safety are minimized.

MAINTAINING THE RELATIONSHIP

As important as it is to deal with all the practical issues, maintaining a close and comfortable relationship is a priority as well. Obviously a relationship is a two-way street, requiring the efforts of both partners, but here are some tips to help support partners do their part:

■ **Communication**—Establishing and maintaining effective communication is important for every relationship. And while communication is a real buzzword these days—making it sound as though it's easy and everyone should be able to do it—the key components of effective communication can be challenging for even the closest of couples. The reality is that the expression of thoughts and feelings comes more naturally to some people than to others, which means that one person in a couple might find it a lot easier to have a heart-to-heart conversation than the other person. In addition, communication takes many different forms, including talking, tone of voice, facial expression, touch, body language, behavior, e-mail/texting, and so on. This means that in one way or another, people are conveying messages to each other virtually all of the time, whether they mean to or not.

■ **Communicating effectively**—Given that communication is going on all the time, it's important to be mindful of what is conveyed to the other person. Ideally, participants in every important conversation will:
  • Accurately convey their ideas, feelings, and needs
  • Respect the ideas, feelings, and needs of the other person
  • Send a clear, unambiguous message
  • Invite (rather than discourage) a response
  • Allow the other person time to respond

While most would agree that all of these are important, the complexities of daily life—particularly in the face of a variable and unpredictable disease like MS—can make even simple interactions feel frustrating or unsatisfying.

Challenges Related to Communication

■ Lack of time in the course of a busy day or week
■ Lack of a quiet, non-distracting place to talk without interruptions

(continued)

Challenges Related to Communication (*continued*)

■ Difficulty putting complex feelings and thoughts into words

■ Concerns about upsetting the other person

■ Embarrassment when talking about certain topics

■ Avoidance of painful or scary issues

■ Memory and attention problems that make it difficult for the person with MS to keep up with the conversation or remember it

■ Mood changes in either partner, including depression, anxiety, or moodiness that get in the way

Sometimes just talking about this list of challenges helps couples pinpoint the particular obstacles they are facing. By bringing attention to them, they can begin to identify strategies to overcome them. For example, some couples decide to have one "date night" every week or two in order to ensure that they have a time and place for good conversation. If the partner with MS is experiencing cognitive changes that get in the way, the support partner can acknowledge this by having important conversations in a distraction-free place, slowing the pace to allow time for the other person to process the information and formulate a response, and checking to make sure that the person has heard and understood the information. When important topics are too difficult or painful to talk about, couples can work with a counselor to help start the process.

Some simple strategies for effective conversations include:

■ Making time for talking.

■ Acknowledging and accepting differences in coping/communication styles.

■ Starting sentences with "I feel . . . I think . . . I need." Sentences starting with "You . . . " tend to sound accusatory and have a tendency to put the other person on the defensive.

■ Giving the other person time to think about what's been said and formulate a response—even if this takes time.

■ Giving clear messages. No matter how much people love each other, they cannot read each other's minds.

Behaviors that interfere with communication include:

■ Over generalizing with statements like "You *always* . . . " or "You *never* . . . " tends to put the other person on the defensive and doesn't allow room for negotiation.

■ Sarcasm can be demeaning and demoralizing.

Listening is as important to an effective conversation as talking; unfortunately, most of us are much better talkers than listeners. Strategies for good listening include:

■ Listening actively and confirming what's been heard; active listening helps avoid confusion and misunderstanding.

■ Paying attention to one's body language; eye-rolling, smirking, finger-jabbing, or answering a cell phone convey as much meaning as your words.

■ Resisting the impulse to interrupt, jump to conclusions, or finish the other person's sentence; patience conveys interest and respect.

■ Asking questions when the other person's meaning or message is confusing; questions demonstrate interest and caring.

■ Letting the other person know if time is needed to think through what's been said and formulate a response; giving notice of the intent to respond is critically important because silence is easily misinterpreted as lack of interest or not caring.

■ Using "ouch" as a short-hand signal when a painful or hurtful statement has been made. "Ouch" is a word that everyone understands. Saying it out loud gives the other person an opportunity to apologize or clarify if no pain was intended, or re-phrase the important message in a less hurtful way.

Acknowledging the challenges to effective communication is the first step; recognizing that each person's feelings and thoughts are valid and deserving of being heard is the second; practicing new ways to maintain communication rather than shutting it down is the third. And seeking help—if needed—from a counselor or other mental health professional to get the tough conversations started, is the fourth.

■ **Maintaining the connection**—MS—the "third wheel"—has a habit of getting in the way. Similar to the way that new babies and growing children can challenge a couple's efforts to enjoy each other's company, MS can as well. Fatigue and other MS symptoms can disrupt plans and diminish both partners' enjoyment of shared activities. Everything takes more planning and preparation, sending spontaneity right out the window. Support partners often find that nothing is simple anymore; everything takes more time, more patience, and more energy. Given these challenges, couples need to work extra hard to maintain their connection and create positive, satisfying opportunities to spend time together.

■ **Shared activities**—When and if the MS progresses, support partners may find that they and their loved ones are able to enjoy fewer and fewer activities together. Suddenly, daily life has been taken over by work, chores, and other responsibilities, with none of the social or recreational outlets they used to share. For many couples this is not just a loss of fun, but a loss of one more aspect of the relationship that bound them together. Working together to keep the fun in life is essential to every relationship.

  • As MS symptoms begin to get in the way of shared activities, couples tend gradually to stop doing them. Over time, their opportunities for shared fun become fewer and fewer, sometimes disappearing entirely. The challenge for couples is to find new ways to do the old, familiar activities or discover new activities they have never tried before. This is a learning process that begins with letting go of the "old way." Like other losses, the letting go often involves a grieving process for both partners.

    Occupational therapists offer suggestions for ways to adapt a shared activity in order to make it possible for the person with MS.

  • Sometimes, a small change can make all the difference. Support partners find it very difficult to slow down enough for their loved one. Walking "in slow motion" is difficult and fatiguing for someone who doesn't have MS. Constantly being on alert to catch someone who trips or falls can take the pleasure out of any shared activity. And having someone—even a beloved person—holding on to one's arm for an entire day or evening can feel exhausting and stifling. Support partners have the right to ask the person with MS to use a mobility aid for shared activities. Sometimes a cane or motorized scooter can make the difference between no outing and a wonderful, satisfying one. And when the activity is finished, the person with MS can put the mobility aid away if she or he chooses.

- Many couples have discovered adaptive sports like swimming, boating, biking, skiing, tennis, and golf. Motorized scooters make long walks or hikes possible, as well as trips to parks, museums, and shopping malls. An RV—either rented or purchased—makes long-distance driving a pleasure, free of worries about the location of the next rest area. With the help of a knowledgeable travel agent, accessible vacations all over the world become a reality.
- Couples also have the opportunity to explore new interests or hobbies together—and many are excited to discover how much fun they can have. Reading, taking classes, playing cards or other games, doing puzzles, and cooking are just a few examples of activities that can be adapted in ways that provide enjoyment for both members of the couple.

The common theme in all of these activities is time spent sharing a common activity that provides enjoyment and opportunities for conversation and interaction. While watching TV together can also provide enjoyment and opportunities for a cuddle, it tends to interfere with conversation. Spending time on computers and iPhones generally offers no connection whatsoever. So couples need to take a careful look at their activities to ensure that they are doing enough to maintain their connectedness.

- **Maintaining relationships with friends and family**—Many support partners report that as the MS progresses, socializing with others becomes increasingly difficult. MS fatigue and other unpredictable symptoms make planning difficult—people's homes aren't accessible, and friends and family may distance themselves. "You really learn who your friends are when MS comes along. Everyone else just seemed to disappear when things got tougher," is a comment often heard from support partners.

In general, people don't disappear because they are mean or uncaring. Most just don't know what to say or how to act in the face of progressive disability. Their awkwardness causes them to withdraw little by little. Support partners may need to take the lead in maintaining these important connections. Strategies might include inviting people over and ordering dinner in if cooking isn't an option, or arranging for an outing to an accessible restaurant or theater. Explaining the unpredictability of MS to others is also very important; they will understand and accept the need for a rain check more easily if they have some familiarity with the disease. And support partners should consider keeping some of those dates even if the person with MS doesn't feel up to it. At first glance this may seem selfish or uncaring, but it is important for support partners to maintain those connections for themselves and for the couple. It's much harder for friends and family to withdraw when periodic contact is maintained.

■ Intimacy is all about connectedness, communication, partnership, and trust. This entire chapter is about finding ways to maintain and nourish intimacy. Sexual expression, which is an important component of intimacy, can be compromised in many ways by MS. Support partners are often puzzled, frustrated, saddened, and frightened by changes in the sexual relationship with their spouse or partner ("Did I do something wrong? . . . Doesn't she love me anymore? . . . Is there someone else?"). A basic understanding of the ways that MS can affect sexuality can be reassuring and helpful. It is helpful to discuss issues concerning problems with sexual function and intimacy with someone on the health care team. The provider should be able to answer questions, but time is often a factor. In offices where there is a nurse, it may be helpful to make an appointment with him or her. The conversation is less apt to be rushed and may feel more comfortable. More detailed discussions about MS and sexuality are available in the Recommended Readings section at the end of the chapter.

■ Sexuality can be affected by MS in three major ways:

1. Damage in the central nervous system can cause sexual symptoms just like it causes other symptoms. The most commonly reported changes are problems with arousal (erections in men and lubrication in women) and problems achieving an orgasm.

These changes are neurological; they have nothing to do with "falling out of love" or "losing interest in one's partner."

2. The others symptoms of MS—including fatigue, weakness, pain, stiffness, bladder and bowel problems, problems with attention and concentration, and depression—can interfere with comfortable sexual activity. In addition, many of the medications used to treat these symptoms can interfere with sexual expression.

3. Less tangible things like attitudes about illness and disability,- self-concept, self-confidence, and changes in roles, can affect sexual feelings in both partners. In particular, support partners who are providing a significant amount of hands-on personal care may find it difficult to maintain sexual feelings for their partner.

Like other changes caused by MS, sexual changes need and deserve attention. Too often a kind of "Don't ask, Don't tell" policy gets in the way. People don't discuss it with their doctors and doctors don't bring it up either. Support partners can encourage their spouse or partner to discuss changes with the health care team (A few hints: Nurses tend to be better with this conversation than physicians; medications can help with MS symptoms that get in the way; a little planning and scheduling can help with the fatigue; physical and occupational therapists can offer strategies to manage some of the logistical problems; counselors can help with the emotional issues.). Every couple will find different ways to deal with their sexual relationship; the important thing is that they give it the attention it deserves and don't just let it lapse like an old library card. Physical intimacy—however it is expressed—is important to remaining close and connected as a couple.

■   **Dealing with mood and cognitive issues**—It is important for support partners to be able to recognize these symptoms and understand how they can affect a person's behavior and interfere with everyday activities; without this understanding, mood and cognitive changes can easily be misinterpreted. A person who is depressed can come across as remote, unloving, irritable, and self-absorbed. Someone who has problems remembering new information, is slow to process information, or has difficulty focusing attention, may seem disinterested, uncaring, or in another world. Support partners may begin to feel abandoned, worried that their loved one has lost interest or found someone else.

- "This isn't the person I married" expresses a fairly common—and profound—sense of loss on the part of support partners. And ironically, it is much less often related to the physical symptoms of MS than with the emotional and cognitive ones. Couples find a variety of ways to work around the physical changes that MS can bring, and most continue to connect emotionally even in the face of significant physical changes. But mood and cognitive changes seem to impact a couple's relationship in a more basic way, affecting the very core of their ties to one another.

- Early recognition and treatment of these problems not only provide relief for the person with MS, but also for the relationship. Depression, irritability, and other mood changes respond well to treatment, which is most often a combination of counseling, medication if needed, and exercise. All have been shown to improve mood in people with MS. While there is no medication to treat cognitive dysfunction, it is important to identify the specific functions that have been affected so that the person (and family members) can learn and implement strategies and work-arounds to compensate for any changes that have occurred. Most importantly, a shared recognition of the problems, whether they are emotional or cognitive, can allow couples to talk openly about them, problem-solve together, and regain the connection they may have temporarily lost as a result of these symptoms.

- **Maintaining balance in the relationship**—When MS symptoms—physical, cognitive, or emotional—interfere with a person's ability to carry out some of his or her roles and responsibilities, a shift begins to occur in the relationship. Support partners may find themselves gradually taking on more and more of the household tasks as the person with MS finds them too difficult to do. The result isn't good for either one of the partners. The support partner may come to feel overburdened, exhausted, and overwhelmed while the person with MS gradually begins to feel sidelined. In order for a relationship to be healthy and satisfying, it needs to be balanced, with each person contributing to it and deriving benefit from it. When one person feels he or she is "doing it all" and the other feels he or she "has nothing to contribute," the relationship is out of whack.

- In the event that a support partner needs to take over some of the responsibilities formerly done by the person with MS, it is important for some kind of trade to occur in order for balance to be maintained. Perhaps the person with MS can take over some of the less physically taxing or cognitively challenging tasks that the support partner used to handle. The situation will be different for every couple and every household, but the key is for each person to feel valued and each person to feel like a giver and a receiver in the relationship.

TAKING CARE OF ONE'S OWN HEALTH

This chapter ends where it began. "Put on your own oxygen mask before assisting the person next to you." It is to everyone's benefit—their own and everyone else's—for support partners to pay attention to their own health and wellness. Support partners who worry about "what will happen to my spouse/partner if something happens to me?" can best address that worry by taking good care of themselves and doing the kinds of planning discussed earlier in the chapter.

- **Nurturing the body and soul**—Adequate rest and exercise are essential to good health. Support partners whose sleep is routinely interrupted by their partners (perhaps because of nighttime bladder issues, periodic limb movements, or generally restless sleep) may need to plan one or two nights a week in a separate room for a little catch-up. Building exercise time into the weekly schedule, even if it means bringing in outside help so that the support partner can get to the gym, is well worth the investment; exercise is good for the body and the mind. Hobbies, time with friends, and attending to one's spiritual needs are all part of a healthy lifestyle, and one can't experience wellness or be an effective support partner without them. Preventive health care is also part of the deal. Support partners can be so preoccupied with their loved one's doctor visits that they forget their own. A regular physical, including the screening tests that are appropriate for one's age group, can catch a

147

problem early. Unfortunately, a loved one's MS is not preventative against illness or disability in the support partner.

- **Paying attention to one's mood**—Support partners are also at risk of depression. Feeling overwhelmed and out of control can lay the foundation, and neglecting one's own needs contributes further. Support partners who find themselves feeling chronically blue or irritable, unable to fall asleep or stay asleep—or, sleeping way too much, having no interest or enjoyment in life, drinking too much, or engaging in other unhealthy behaviors, need to discuss it with their health care provider. These are not signs of weakness—they are possible indications of significant depression, particularly if they continue without relief for weeks at a time. The responsibilities of a support partner are challenging enough without trying to manage them under the painful weight of depression; depression makes everything look and feel harder.

- **Heeding the warning signs**—Even the kindest and most loving person can reach a limit. Feelings of sadness, frustration, and impatience that have spun out of control can be expressed in all kinds of ways—cruel words, rough handling when helping a person with activities of daily living, or even disappearing for hours or days at a time. Support partners need to pay attention if they find themselves behaving in ways they wouldn't want others to see. These are signals of emotional overload. Support partners can and should reach out for help at these times. There is no need for shame or embarrassment—overload can happen to anyone, regardless of age, gender, ethnicity, education, or socioeconomic status. The National MS Society can help support partners access the support and community services they need to get the situation back to a more manageable level.

Support for the support partner is central to the Can Do MS philosophy. When a loved one is diagnosed with MS, the support partner lives with it as well. It is our hope that this chapter provides the encouragement support partners need to pay adequate attention to their own health and wellness.

RECOMMENDED READING

Booklets available from the National Multiple Sclerosis Society (at www.
nationalmssociety.org/brochures or by calling 1-800-344-4867): *A Guide
for Caregivers Hiring Help at Home: The Basic Facts.*
Miller, D., & Crawford, P. (2005). The Caregiving Relationship. In R. Kalb (Ed.)
Multiple Sclerosis: A Guide for Families (3rd ed.). New York: Demos
Health.
Miller, D., & Kalb, R. (2012). How Multiple Sclerosis Affects the Family. In R. Kalb
(Ed.) *Multiple Sclerosis: The Questions You Have, The Answers You Need*
(5th ed.). New York: Demos Health.

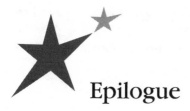

Epilogue

YOU *CAN* LIVE FULLY WITH MS

Everything we do at Can Do MS is driven by one simple belief: you are more than your MS. Our vision, mission, and core values are rooted in the legacy and belief of our founder, Jimmie Heuga, that everyone living with MS has the power to live full lives. Reading this book is the start of a whole new way of thinking about and living with multiple sclerosis.

LIVING FULLY WITH MS INVOLVES MORE THAN WELLNESS: IT INVOLVES EVALUATION OF LIFE STRATEGIES

The incurable nature of MS combined with the complexity of its various stages, its individual nature, and its unpredictability, create multi-faceted challenges for people living with MS and their loved ones. Lifestyle empowerment is about learning the individualized skills and mindset to take charge of your health and your life with MS.

APPLYING THESE STRATEGIES IS A WHOLE NEW WAY OF LOOKING AT MS

Our whole person, whole health, and whole community approach to MS provides people with MS and their support partners a deeper and broader understanding of their unique condition. Exploring the physical, interpersonal, emotional, intellectual, and spiritual aspects of living with MS helps them gain more in-depth understanding of their MS, their general health, and themselves. It blends that knowledge with realistic and personalized goal setting, and helps people learn what is possible with MS and how to live fuller, richer lives within the constraints of MS.

TODAY IS THE START OF YOUR CAN DO JOURNEY

Now that you have been introduced to a whole new way of thinking about and living with MS, either as a person with the disease or the support partner of that person, it is time to make a promise to yourself and a commitment to the future. We suggest framing that promise this way:

I AM more than my MS
I CAN see beyond the challenges of MS
I WILL realize what is possible living with MS

Your own promise may look entirely different. The importance of making this promise is that it encourages you to "look outside the box" of living with MS and to see a different future. Making this promise will assist you in considering positive life changes and empower you to make those changes.

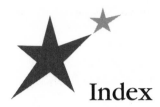

Index

distress of, 44
MS as challenges/threat, 27–29
Physiatrists, 20
Physical activity, US Surgeon
   General's Report on, 83–84
Physical function, 85
Physical therapists (PT), 20–21, 83,
   88, 94, 100
   suggestion from, 94
Physician assistants (PA), 20
Pilates, 88
Plans
   goals versus, 5–6
   making, 6
   SMART, 7–8
Polyunsaturated fats, 108
Power pantry, 107
Practical issues
   financial worries, 133–134
   future care needs, 134
   providing care, 132–133
   quality of life, 135–138
Pre-contemplation stage, 3
Preparation stage, 4
Primary health care provider, 19
Problem-solving skills, in
   patients, 44
Pseudobulbar affect (PBA), laughing
   and crying, 54
Psychiatrists, 21
PT, *See* Physical therapists

Quality of life, 132
   maintaining, 135–138
   recreational activities, 135

Range of Motion (ROM), 97–98
Rating of Perceived Exertion scale
   (RPE), 89, 90
Realistic plan, 8
Recreational activities, 135

Registered Dietician (RD), 21
Registered nurses (RN), 20
Relationship maintenance, 138–147
   with friends and family
   balance, 146–147
   mood and cognitive issues,
      145–147
   sexuality symptoms, 144–145
Resilience, 126–127
RN, *See* Registered nurses
ROM, *See* Range of Motion
RPE, *See* Rating of Perceived
   Exertion scale

Sadness and loss, 130
Self efficacy, 125–126
Self-help groups, 52
Self-monitoring, 9
Sensory symptoms, medications,
   76–77
Sexual dysfunction, in MS, 80
Sleep disorders, 124–125
SLP, *See* Speech/language
   pathologist
SMART plan, 7–8
Smoking, effects of, 123
Social workers, 21, 55
Someday stage, *See* Contemplation
   stage
Soon stage, *See* Preparation
   stage
Spasticity, 69, 71, 76, 77, 97
Specific plan, 7
Speech/language pathologist
   (SLP), 21
Spirituality, 126–127
Stress, 13–14, 74, 78, 130, 138
   anxiety stems, 132, 134
   management, 43
Sunshine vitamin, 110
Support groups, 21–22